AF522094

HOSPITAL, NURSING AND HEALTH CARE

HOSPITAL, NURSING AND HEALTH CARE

Ravish Verma

CENTRUM PRESS
NEW DELHI-110002 (INDIA)

CENTRUM PRESS
H.O.: 4360/4, Ansari Road, Daryaganj,
New Delhi-110002 (India)
Tel: 23278000, 23261597, 23255577, 23286875

B.O.: No. 1015, Ist Main Road, BSK IIIrd Stage,
IIIrd Phase, IIIrd Block, Bangalore-560085 (INDIA)
Tel: 080-41723429

Email: centrumpress@gmail.com
Visit us at: www.centrumpress.com

Hospital, Nursing and Health Care

First Edition, 2010

ISBN 978-93-80540-88-7

PRINTED IN INDIA

Printed at Balaji Offset, Delhi.

Contents

Preface

A hospital is an institution for health care providing patient treatment by specialized staff and equipment, and often, but not always providing for longer-term patient stays. Today, hospitals usually are funded by the public sector, by health organizations, (for profit or nonprofit), health insurance companies or charities, including by direct charitable donations. In history, however, hospitals often were founded and funded by religious orders or charitable individuals and leaders. Similarly, modern-day hospitals are largely staffed by professional physicians, surgeons, and nurses, whereas in history, this work usually was performed by the founding religious orders or by volunteers. The best-known type of hospital is the general hospital, which is set up to deal with many kinds of disease and injury, and typically has an emergency department to deal with immediate and urgent threats to health.

Nursing is a healthcare profession focused on the care of individuals, families, and communities so they may attain, maintain, or recover optimal health and quality of life from birth to death. Nurses work in a large variety of specialties where they work independently and as part of a team to assess, plan, implement and evaluate care. The authority for the practice of nursing is based upon a social contract that delineates professional rights and responsibilities as well as mechanisms for public accountability. In almost all countries, nursing practice is defined and governed by law, and entrance to the profession is regulated at national or state level.

Health care, or healthcare, is the treatment and management of illness, and the preservation of health through services offered by the medical, dental, complementary and alternative medicine, pharmaceutical, clinical sciences (*in vitro* diagnostics), nursing, and allied health professions. Health care embraces all the goods and services designed to promote health, including "preventive, curative and palliative interventions, whether directed to individuals or to populations". The definition of health care is continuously evolving and varies significantly between different cultures.

The book provides readers with an introductory overview of basic issues related to hospital, nursing and health care. Various facets of issues related to health care and nursing industry and services are covered in detail.

—Dr. Ravish Verma

1

Introduction

Health Care

Health care, or health care, is the treatment and management of illness, and the preservation of health through services offered by the medical, dental, complementary and alternative medicine, pharmaceutical, clinical sciences (*in vitro* diagnostics), nursing, and allied health professions. Health care embraces all the goods and services designed to promote health, including "preventive, curative and palliative interventions, whether directed to individuals or to populations". The definition of health care is continuously evolving and varies significantly between different cultures.

Before the term *health care* became popular, English-speakers referred to *medicine* or to the *health sector* and spoke of the treatment and prevention of illness and disease. The social and political issue of access to healthcare in the US has led to public debate and confusing use of terms such as "health care" (medical management of illness or disease), health insurance (reimbursement of health care costs), and the public health (the collective state and range of health in a population).

Healthcare Industry

The delivery of modern health care depends on an expanding group of trained professionals coming together as an interdisciplinary team. The healthcare industry incorporates several sectors that are dedicated to providing services and products dedicated to improving the health of individuals. According to market classifications of industry such as the Global Industry Classification Standard and the Industry Classification Benchmark the healthcare industry includes health care equipment & services and pharmaceuticals, biotechnology & life sciences. The particular sectors associated with these groups are: biotechnology, diagnostic substances, drug delivery, drug manufacturers, hospitals, medical equipment and instruments, diagnostic laboratories, nursing homes, providers of health care plans and home health care.

According to government classifications of Industry, which are mostly based on the United Nations system, the International Standard Industrial Classification, health care generally consists of hospital activities, medical and dental practice activities, and other human health activities. The last class consists of all activities for human health not performed by hospitals or by medical doctors or dentists. This involves activities of, or under the supervision of, nurses, midwives, physiotherapists, scientific or diagnostic laboratiories, pathology clinics, ambulance, nursing home, or other para-medical practitioners in the field of optometry, hydrotherapy, medical massage, music therapy, occupational therapy, speech therapy, chiropody, homeopathy, chiropractice, acupuncture, etc.

Health Care Reforms in the United States

Health care reform is a major agenda in the United States aside economic recovery. President Barack Obama and Democratic leaders of Congress are keen to overhaul the current health care system, citing it as inefficient and unaffordable to Americans, and replace it with a comprehensive national system of health insurance.

In 2009, the overhaul of the health care system in the United States was approved and the Senate passed an $871 billion bill. This was a major step towards health care reform and the stage was now set.

By the end of March 2009, the chairmen of five Congressional committees had reached a consensus on the main ingredients of legislation, and insurance industry representatives had made some major concessions. The chairmen, all Democrats, agreed that everyone must carry insurance and that employers should be required to help pay for it. They also agreed that the government should offer a public health insurance plan as an alternative to private insurance.

But the matter started to become complicated when the Democratic Party lost its Senate seat in Massachusetts to Republicans losing its 60th vote which gave it an advantage over the Republicans. A health care reform was further dealt a blow with the announcement that Billy Tauzin, a top lobbyist who positioned the pharmaceutical industry firmly behind healthcare reform, would resign. A meeting held between Democrat and Republican lawmakers on February 25, 2010, resulted in an impasse.

Research

Top impact factor academic journals in the health care field include *Health Affairs* and *Milbank Quarterly*. The *New England Journal of Medicine, British Medical Journal,* and the *Journal of the American Medical Association* are more general journals.

Biomedical research (or experimental medicine), in general simply known as medical research, is the basic research, applied research, or translational research conducted to aid the body of knowledge in the field of medicine. Medical research can be divided into two general categories: the evaluation of new treatments for both safety and efficacy in what are termed clinical trials, and all other research that contributes to the development of new treatments. The latter is termed preclinical research if its goal is specifically to elaborate knowledge for the development of new therapeutic strategies. A new paradigm to biomedical research is being termed translational research, which focuses on iterative feedback loops between the basic and clinical research domains to accelerate knowledge translation from the bedside to the bench, and back again.

In terms of pharmaceutical R&D spending, Europe spends a little less that the United States (€22.50bn compared to €27.05bn in 2006) and there is less growth in European R&D spending. Pharmaceuticals and other medical devices are the leading high technology exports of Europe and the United States. However, the United States dominates the biopharmaceutical field, accounting for the three quarters of the world's biotechnology revenues and 80% of world R&D spending in biotechnology.

World Health Organization

The World Health Organization (WHO) is a specialized United Nations agency which acts as a coordinator and researcher for public health around the world. Established on 7 April 1948, and headquartered in Geneva, Switzerland, the agency inherited the mandate and resources of its predecessor, the Health Organization, which had been an agency of the League of Nations. The WHO's constitution states that its mission "is the attainment by all peoples of the highest possible level of health."

Its major task is to combat disease, especially key infectious diseases, and to promote the general health of the peoples of the world. Examples of its work include years of fighting smallpox. In 1979 the WHO declared that the disease had been eradicated - the first disease in history to be completely eliminated by deliberate human design. The WHO is nearing success in developing vaccines against malaria and schistosomiasis and aims to eradicate polio within the next few years. The organization has already endorsed the world's first official HIV/AIDS Toolkit for Zimbabwe from October 3, 2006, making it an international standard.

The WHO is financed by contributions from member states and from donors. In recent years the WHO's work has involved more collaboration, currently around 80 such partnerships, with NGOs and the pharmaceutical industry, as well as with foundations such as the Bill and Melinda Gates Foundation and the Rockefeller Foundation. Voluntary contributions to the WHO from national and local governments, foundations and NGOs, other UN organizations, and the private sector (including pharmaceutical companies), now exceed that of assessed contributions (dues) from its 193 member nations.

Economics

Health economics is a branch of economics concerned with issues related to scarcity in the allocation of health and health care. Broadly, health economists study the functioning of the health care system and the private and social causes of health-affecting behaviours such as smoking.

A seminal 1963 article by Kenneth Arrow, often credited with giving rise to the health economics as a discipline, drew conceptual distinctions between health and other goals. Factors that distinguish health economics from other areas include extensive government intervention, intractable uncertainty in several dimensions, asymmetric information, and externalities. Governments tend to regulate the health care industry heavily and also tend to be the largest payer within the market. Uncertainty is intrinsic to health, both in patient outcomes and financial concerns. The knowledge gap that exists between a physician and a patient can prevent the patient from accurately describing his symptoms or enable the physician to prescribe unnecessary but profitable services; these imbalances lead to market failures resulting from asymmetric information. Externalities arise frequently when considering health and health care. notably in the context of infectious disease. For example, making an effort to avoid catching a cold, or practising safer sex, affects people other than the decision maker.

The scope of health economics is neatly encapsulated by Alan William's "plumbing diagram" dividing the discipline into eight distinct topics:

- What influences health? (other than health care)
- What is health and what is its value
- The demand for health care
- The supply of health care
- Micro-economic evaluation at treatment level
- Market equilibrium
- Evaluation at whole system level; and,
- Planning, budgeting and monitoring mechanisms.

Consuming just under 10 percent of gross domestic product of most developed nations, health care can form an enormous part of a country's economy. In 2001, health care consumed 8.4 per cent of GDP across the OECD countries with the United States (13.9%), Switzerland (10.9%), and Germany (10.7%) being the top three.

The United States and Canada account for 48% of world pharmaceutical sales, while Europe, Japan, and all other nations account for 30%, 9%, and 13%, respectively. United States accounts for the three quarters of the world's biotechnology revenues.

Systems

Social health insurance is where a nation's entire population is eligible for health care coverage, and this coverage and the services provided are regulated. In almost every country, state or municipality with a government health care system a parallel private, and usually for-profit, system is allowed to operate. This is sometimes referred to as two-tier health care. The scale, extent, and funding of these private systems is variable.

A traditional view is that improvements in health result from advancements in medical science. The medical model of health focuses on the eradication of illness through diagnosis and effective treatment. In contrast, the social model of health places emphasis on changes that can be made in society and in people's own lifestyles to make the population healthier. It defines *illness* from the point of view of the individual's functioning within their society rather than by monitoring for changes in biological or physiological signs.

The United States currently operates under a mixed market health care system. Government sources (federal, state, and local) account for 45% of U.S. health care expenditures. Private sources account for the remainder of costs, with 38% of people receiving health coverage through their employers and 17% arising from other private payment such as private insurance and out-of-pocket co-pays. Opponents of government intervention into the market generally believe that such intervention distorts pricing as government agents would be operating outside of the corporate model and the principles of market discipline; they have less short and medium-term incentives than private agents to make purchases that can generate revenues and avoid bankruptcy. Health system reform in the United States usually focuses around three suggested systems, with proposals currently underway to integrate these systems in various ways to provide a number of health care options. First is single-payer, a term meant to describe a single agency managing a single system, as found in most modernized countries as well as some states and municipalities within the United States. Second are employer or individual insurance mandates, with which the state of Massachusetts has experimented. Finally, there is consumer-driven health, in which systems, consumers, and patients have more control of how they access care. This is argued to provide a greater incentive to find cost-saving health care approaches. Critics of consumer-driven health say that it would benefit the healthy but be insufficient for the chronically sick, much as the current system operates. Over the past thirty years, most of the nation's health care has moved from the second model operating with not-for-profit institutions to the third model operating with for-profit institutions; the greater problems with this approach have been the gradual deregulation of HMOs resulting in fewer of the promised choices for consumers, and the steady increase in consumer cost that has marginalized consumers and burdened states with excessive urgent health care costs that are avoided with consumers have adequate access to preventive health care.

A few states have taken serious steps toward universal health care coverage, most notably Minnesota, Massachusetts and Connecticut, with recent examples being the Massachusetts 2006 Health Reform Statute and Connecticut's SustiNet plan to provide quality, affordable health care to state residents.

Politics

The politics of health care depends largely on which country one is in. Current concerns in England, for instance, revolve around the use of private finance initiatives to build hospitals which it is argued costs taxpayers more in the long run. In Germany and France, concerns are more based on the rising cost of drugs to the governments. In Brazil, an important political issue is the breach of intellectual property rights, or patents, for the domestic manufacture of antiretroviral drugs used in the treatment of HIV/AIDS.

The South African government, whose population sets the record for HIV infections, came under pressure for its refusal to admit there is any connection with AIDS because of the cost it would have involved. In the United States 12% to 16% of the citizens are still unable to afford health insurance. State boards and the Department of Health regulate inpatient care to reduce the national health care deficit. To tackle the problems of the perpetually increasing number of uninsured, and costs associated with the US health care system, President Barack Obama says he favours the creation of a universal health care system. However, *New York Times* opinion columnist Paul Krugman said that Obama's plan would not actually provide universal coverage, and Factcheck.org alleges that Obama's predicted savings were exaggerated. In contrast, the state of Oregon and the city of San Francisco are both examples of governments that adopted universal healthcare systems for strictly fiscal reasons.

Health Care by Country

Health care systems are composed of individuals and organizations that aim to meet the health care needs of target populations. There are a wide variety of health care systems around the world. In some countries, the health care system planning is distributed among market participants, whereas in others planning is made more centrally among governments, trade unions, charities, religious, or other co-ordinated bodies to deliver planned health care services targeted to the populations they serve. However, health care planning has often been evolutionary rather than revolutionary.

Hospital, Health Care and Nursing

A hospital is an institution for health care providing patient treatment by specialized staff and equipment, and often, but not always providing for longer-term patient stays.

Today, hospitals usually are funded by the public sector, by health organizations, (for profit or nonprofit), health insurance companies or charities, including by direct charitable donations. In history, however, hospitals often were founded and funded by religious orders or charitable individuals and leaders. Similarly, modern-day hospitals are largely staffed by professional physicians, surgeons, and nurses, whereas in history, this work usually was performed by the founding religious orders or by volunteers.

Etymology

During the Middle Ages the hospital could serve other functions, such as almshouse for the poor, hostel for pilgrims, or hospital school. The name comes from Latin *hospes* (host), which also is the root for the English words *hospice, hotel, hostel,* and *hospitality*. The modern word *hotel* derives from the French word *hostel,* which featured a silent, eventually removed from the word to leave a circumflex on modern French *hotel*. The word also is related to the German word 'Spital'.

Grammar of the word differs slightly depending on the dialect. In the U.S., *hospital* usually requires an article; in Britain and elsewhere, the word normally is used without an article when it is the object of a preposition and when referring to a patient ("in/ to the hospital" vs. "in/to hospital"); in Canada, both uses are found.

Types

Some patients go to a hospital just for diagnosis, treatment, or therapy and then leave ('outpatients') without staying overnight; while others are 'admitted' and stay overnight or for several weeks or months ('inpatients'). Hospitals usually are distinguished from other types of medical facilities by their ability to admit and care for inpatients and the others often are described as a clinic.

General

The best-known type of hospital is the general hospital, which is set up to deal with many kinds of disease and injury, and typically has an emergency department to deal with immediate and urgent threats to health. A general hospital typically is the major health care facility in its region, with large numbers of beds for intensive care and long-term care; and specialized facilities for surgery, plastic surgery, childbirth, bioassay laboratories, and so forth. Larger cities may have many several hospitals of varying sizes and facilities. Some hospitals, especially in the United States, have their own ambulance service.

Specialized

Types of specialized hospitals include trauma centres,

rehabilitation hospitals, children's hospitals, seniors' (geriatric) hospitals, and hospitals for dealing with specific medical needs such as psychiatric problems, certain disease categories, and so forth.

A hospital may be a single building or a number of buildings on a campus. Many hospitals with pre-twentieth-century origins began as one building and evolved into campuses. Some hospitals are affiliated with universities for medical research and the training of medical personnel such as physicians and nurses, often called teaching hospitals. Worldwide, most hospitals are run on a nonprofit basis by governments or charities. Within the United States, most hospitals are nonprofit.

Teaching

A teaching hospital combines assistance to patients with teaching to medical students and nurses and often is linked to a medical school or nursing school. Some of these are associated with universities.

Clinics

A medical facility smaller than a hospital is generally called a clinic, and often is run by a government agency for health services or a private partnership of physicians (in nations where private practice is allowed). Clinics generally provide only outpatient services.

Departments

Hospitals vary widely in the services they offer and therefore, in the departments they have. They may have acute services such as an emergency department or specialist trauma centre, burn unit, surgery, or urgent care. These may then be backed up by more specialist units such as cardiology or coronary care unit, intensive care unit, neurology, cancer centre, and obstetrics and gynecology.

Some hospitals will have outpatient departments and some will have chronic treatment units such as behavioural health services, dentistry, dermatology, psychiatric ward, rehabilitation services, and physical therapy.

Common support units include a dispensary or pharmacy, pathology, and radiology, and on the non-medical side, there often are medical records departments and/or release of information department.

Acute Assessment Unit

An acute assessment unit, or acute admissions unit, (AAU) is a short-stay department in UK hospitals that is sometimes part of the emergency department, although a separate department. The AAU acts as a gateway between a patient's general practitioner, the emergency department, and the wards of the hospital. The AAU helps the emergency department produce a healthy turnaround for patients, helping with the four-hour waiting rule.

An AAU is usually made up of several bays and has a small number of side-rooms and treatment rooms. They are fully equipped with emergency medical treatment facilities including defibrilators and resuscitation equipment.

Patients

From the emergency department, patients can be moved to AAU where they will undergo further tests and stabilisation before they are transferred to the relevant ward or sent home. Also, patients can be admitted straight to AAU from their general practitioner if he or she believes the patient needs hospital treatment. A patient's stay in the unit is limited, usually no more than 48 hours.

The AAU deals with admissions only, patients will never be transferred from a ward to the AAU. Surgical Procedures are not carried out in the unit either; these are referred on to the relevant theatre such as cardiothoracics and general surgery.

Staff

Senior staff in an AAU include a consultant in general medicine, emergency medicine, or critical care. Often a registrar in general medicine, and a ward sister or a charge nurse have roles in the unit. A number of staff nurses work alongside the senior staff to provide care to patients in the unit.

Although AAU has its own staff trained to deal with patients and provide care, members of staff from other departments in the hospital are needed in AAU to assess patients and provide further diagnosis. Typical examples of staff who may be needed in AAU are general surgeons, cardiothoracic surgeons, cardiologists, and a psychiatric liaison nurse.

Alternative Names for the Department

Different hospitals use different names for the department - common names for this department are:

- Acute Assessment Unit
- Acute Admissions Unit
- Clinical Decision Unit (CDU)
- Medical Assessment Unit (MAU)
- Multi speciality Assessment Area (MSAA)
- Medical Receiving Unit (MRU)
- Emergency Receiving Unit (ERU).

Coronary Care Unit

A coronary care unit (CCU) is a hospital ward specialized in the care of patients with heart attacks, unstable angina and (in practice) various other cardiac conditions that require continuous monitoring and treatment.

Characteristics

The main feature of coronary care is the availability of telemetry or the continuous monitoring of the cardiac rhythm by electrocardiography. This allows early intervention with medication, cardioversion or defibrillation, improving the prognosis.

As arrhythmias are relatively common in this group, patients with myocardial infarction or unstable angina are routinely admitted to the coronary care unit. For other indications, such as atrial fibrillation, a specific indication is generally necessary, while for others, such as heart block, coronary care unit admission is standard.

Local Differences

In the United States, coronary care units are usually subsets of intensive care units (ICU) dedicated to the care of critically ill cardiac patients. These units are usually present in hospitals that routine engage in cardiothoracic surgery. Invasive monitoring such as with pulmonary artery catheters is common, as are supportive modalities such as mechanical ventilation and intra-aortic balloon pumps (IABP).

Certain hospitals, such as Johns Hopkins, maintain mixed units consisting of both Acute care units for the critically ill, and intermediate care units for patients who are not critical.

Acute Coronary Care

Acute coronary care units (ACCU), also called "critical coronary care units" (CCCU) is equivalent to intensive care in the level of service provided. Patients with acute myocardial infarction, cardiogenic shock, or post-operative "open-heart" patients commonly abide here.

Subacute Coronary Care

Subacute coronary care units (SCCU), also called Progressive care units (PCU), Intermediate coronary care units (ICCU), or stepdown units, and provide a level of care intermediate to that of the intensive care unit and that of the general medical floor. These units typically serve patients who require cardiac telemetry such as those with unstable angina.

Coronary care units developed in the 1960s when it became clear that close monitoring by specially trained staff, cardiopulmonary resuscitation and medical measures could reduce the mortality from complications of cardiovascular disease. The first description of a CCU was given in 1961 to the British Thoracic Society, and early CCUs were located in Sydney, Kansas City and Philadelphia. Studies published in 1967 revealed that those observed in a coronary care setting had consistently better outcomes. The first coronary care unit was opened at Bethany Medical Centre in Kansas City, Kansas by Dr. Hugh Day, and he coined the term. Bethany Medical Centre is also where the first "crash carts" were developed.

Emergency Department

The Emergency Department (ED), sometimes termed Accident & Emergency (A&E), Emergency Room (ER), Emergency Ward (EW), or Casualty Department is a hospital or primary care department that provides initial treatment to patients with a broad spectrum of illnesses and injuries, some of which may be life-threatening and require immediate attention. In some countries, Emergency Departments have become important entry points for those without other means of access to medical care. Staff teams treat emergency patients and provide support to family members. The emergency departments of most hospitals operate around the clock, although staffing levels attempt to mirror patient volume, which in most ED's finds its nadir between 2:00 am and 6:00 am. Most patients seek the Emergency Department in the afternoon and evening hours, and staffing mirrors this phenomenon.

History

The first specialized trauma care centre in the world was opened in 1911 in the United States at the University of Louisville Hospital in Louisville, Kentucky, and was developed by surgeon Arnold Griswold during the 1930s. Griswold also equipped police and fire vehicles with medical supplies and trained officers to give emergency care while en route to the hospital.

Department Layout

A typical emergency department has several different areas, each specialized for patients with particular severities or types of illness.

In the *triage* area, patients are seen by an RN or LPN, who completes a preliminary evaluation, before they are transferred to another area of the ED or a different department in the hospital. One body of expertise that seems particularly applicable to emergency medicine services is Operations Management. Operations management utilizes a systems approach to the provision of a service, including the definition of the particular characteristics of a service (such as the service package, the service process, and the virtual value chain embedded in that service), structured planning for service quality, appropriate service metrics, selected management tools, and consideration of strategies for interdisciplinary collaboration, as well as cultural change. The *resuscitation* area is a key ultimately, the value of an operations management approach to management of the ED is explicit consideration of all salient elements of the service process in a systematic manner.

In doing so, it is important to link clearly the service function to the institutions mission/strategic plan, as well as the expectations and needs of ED patients who are served there. They are sent to the *minors* area. Such patients may still have been found to have significant problems, including fractures, dislocations, and lacerations requiring suturing.

Asplin (A Conceptual Model of Emergency Department Crowding. Ann Emerg Med. 2003; 42:173-180), describes a three-phase "input – throughput – output" model of emergency services. This model is applicable to the challenge and solutions to the problem of ED overcrowding that has occurred in many communities in the US.

The information paper includes the following sections:

Some departments employ a *play therapist* whose job is to put children at ease to reduce the anxiety caused by visiting the emergency department, as well as provide distraction therapy for simple procedures.

Many hospitals have a separate area for evaluation of psychiatric problems. These are often staffed by psychiatrists and mental health nurses and social workers. There is typically at least one room for people who are actively a risk to themselves or others (e.g. suicidal).

Intangibility: Services are not manufactured according to precise standards, nor can they be stored. How consumers perceive services is very subjective, since they are a performance rather than a tangible good. Variability: Consistent service delivery is very difficult, particularly in fields such as medicine, due to the high labour contribution of the service along with the variation between clinicians. Inseparability: Service quality is extremely difficult to control since it is produced and consumed at the same time. There is no opportunity to measure or inspect the service prior to actually delivering it. Additionally, the consumer (patient) significantly impacts the quality of the service provided. For example, the description of a patient's symptoms can significantly affect the outcome of the visit. The better the description, the more likely a better outcome.

Signage

A hospital with an emergency department usually has prominent signage reading *Emergency* or *Accident and Emergency* (often in white text on a red background) and an arrow to indicate where patients should proceed. Some American states closely regulate the design and content of such signs and require wording such as "Comprehensive Emergency Medical Service" and "Physician On Duty", to prevent persons in need of critical care from presenting to facilities that are not fully equipped and staffed.

Nomenclature

In Australia and Canada, the department is usually referred to as the *Emergency Department* or *Emerg.*

In the United Kingdom, New Zealand, Hong Kong, Singapore, and Ireland specifically, the department is known as *A&E* (Accident & Emergency). In response to the number of 'minor' injuries that are often presented within the department, some hospitals now choose to only use the term *ED* (Emergency Department) in order to emphasise urgent cases only. Despite this, all road signs to the department throughout the UK read *A&E,* and this remains unchanged. Most teaching hospitals and district general hospitals (DGHs) have an A&E department. The largest such department in the UK is in the city of Leicester (Leicester Royal Infirmary). The term *Casualty,* which preceded A&E in the UK (and is still at times informally used to denote the emergency department of a hospital) is no longer considered appropriate by emergency medical staff in the United Kingdom and Ireland, for similar aforementioned reasons.

In the United States an emergency department is often referred to by both laypeople and medical professionals as an *emergency room* or an "ER." [Medical professionals occasionally call it whatever its name is within their specific hospitals, or simply "emergency."] The term "emergency room" is based on historic usage and is a misnomer today, for a modern hospital's emergency facilities do not consist of only a single room. The ER interacts with every other department in the hospital and often represents a significant percentage of the hospital's work load and finances.

During the 1990s, an effort began to change to the more accurate term *emergency department* (ED), which is a term increasingly used by members of the specialty internationally. The updated name has not yet caught on to the mainstream American public, perhaps due in part to the popularity of the TV show *ER*, and the heavy marketing of the abbreviation "ED" for erectile dysfunction by pharmaceutical companies. However, the term does have wide circulation among emergency medicine staff. Individual hospitals may also refer to the department by different names, such as emergency ward, emergency centre, emergency unit, etc.

Leading journals, including the Annals of Emergency Medicine, published by the American College of Emergency Physicians, and the Emergency Medicine Journal (emj) of the British Association for Emergency Medicine (BAEM), consistently use the term *emergency department*.

In some countries, including the United States, Europe and Canada, a smaller facility that may provide assistance in medical emergencies is known as a clinic. Larger communities often have walk-in clinics where people with medical problems that would not be considered serious enough to warrant an emergency department visit can be seen. These clinics often do not operate on a 24 hour basis.

The term "urgency" instead of "emergency" is used in some Latin American countries. Emergency departments are known as *"servicios de urgencia"* and they function in a similar fashion to European emergency departments.

United States

Many U.S. emergency rooms are exceedingly busy. A survey of New York area doctors in February 2007 found that injuries and even deaths have been caused by excessive waits for hospital beds by ER patients. A 2005 patient survey found an average ER wait time from 2.3 hours in Iowa to 5.0 hours in Arizona.

One inspection of Los Angeles area hospitals by Congressional staff found the ERs operating at an average of 116% of capacity (meaning there were more patients than available treatment spaces) with insufficient beds to accommodate victims of a terrorist attack the size of the 2004 Madrid train bombings. Three of the five Level I trauma centres were on "diversion", meaning ambulances with all but the most severely injured patients were being directed elsewhere because the ER could not safely accommodate any more patients. This controversial practice was banned in Massachusetts (except for major incidents, such as a fire in the ER), effective January 1, 2009; in response, hospitals have devoted more staff to the ER at peak times and moved some elective procedures to non-peak times.

United Kingdom

All A&E departments throughout the United Kingdom are financed and managed by the NHS of each constituent country (England, Scotland, Wales and Northern Ireland). As with most other NHS services, emergency care is provided to all, both resident citizens and those not ordinarily resident in the UK, free at the point of need and regardless of any ability to pay.

Historically, waits for assessment in A&E were very long in some areas of the UK. In October 2002, the Department of Health introduced a four-hour target in emergency departments that required departments to assess and treat patients within four hours of arrival, with referral and assessment by other departments if deemed necessary. Present policy is that 98% of all patient cases do not "breach" this four-hour wait.

The 4-hour target triggered the introduction of the acute assessment unit (also known as the medical assessment unit), which works alongside the emergency department but is outside it for statistical purposes in the bed management cycle. It is claimed that though A&E targets have resulted in significant improvements in completion times, the current target would not have been possible without some form of patient re-designation or re-labelling taking place, so true improvements are somewhat less than headline figures might suggest and it is doubtful that a single target (fitting all A&E and related services) is sustainable.

Patient Experience

If the patient's service expectation is not met, there are ways to remedy this shortcoming. Service recovery is an effective tool to prevent patient defection, but it is necessary to have a well crafted plan in place before the actual event occurs. Patient retention can have a significant financial impact.

Patients are becoming more sophisticated and the healthcare industry must take notice of this. Other sectors of the economy are providing an ever higher quality of service and are raising consumers' expectations along with it. If budget motels, low cost airlines and quick auto lube outlets can produce consistently high quality service encounters, patients will only come to expect that much and more from high-tech and high-cost medical encounters.

Critical Conditions Handled

Cardiac Arrest

Cardiac arrest may occur in the ED/A&E or a patient may be transported by ambulance to the emergency department already in this state. Treatment is basic life support and advanced life support as taught in advanced life support and advanced cardiac life support courses. This is an immediately life-threatening condition which requires immediate action in salvageable cases.

Heart Attack

Patients arriving to the emergency department with a myocardial infarction (heart attack) are likely to be triaged to the resuscitation area. They will receive oxygen and monitoring and have an early ECG; aspirin will be given if not contraindicated or not already administered by the ambulance team; morphine or diamorphine will be given for pain; sub lingual (under the tongue) or buccal (between cheek and upper gum) glyceryl trinitrate [nitroglycerin] (GTN or NTG) will be given, unless contraindicated by the presence of other drugs, such as drugs that treat erectile dysfunction.

An ECG that reveals ST segment elevation or new left bundle branch block suggests complete blockage of one of the main coronary arteries. These patients require immediate reperfusion (re-opening) of the occluded vessel. This can be achieved in two ways: [thrombolysis] (clot-busting medication) or percutaneous transluminal coronary angioplasty (PTCA). Both of these are effective in reducing significantly the mortality of myocardial infarction. Many centres are now moving to the use of PTCA as it is somewhat more effective than thrombolysis if it can be administered early. This may involve transfer to a nearby facility with facilities for angioplasty.

Trauma

Major trauma, the term for patients with multiple injuries, often from a road traffic accident or a fall, is treated by a trauma team who have been trained using the principles taught in the internationally recognized Advanced Trauma Life Support (ATLS) course of the American College of Surgeons. Some other international training bodies have started to run similar courses based on the same principles.

The services that are provided in an emergency department can range from simple x-rays and the setting of broken bones to those of a full-scale trauma centre. A patient's chance of survival is greatly improved if the patient receives definitive treatment (i.e. surgery or reperfusion) within one hour of an accident (such as a car accident) or onset of acute illness (such as a heart attack). This critical time frame is commonly known as the "golden hour."

Some emergency departments in smaller hospitals are located near a helipad which is used by helicopters to transport a patient to a trauma centre. This inter-hospital transfer is often done when a patient requires advanced medical care unavailable at the local facility. In such cases the emergency department can only stabilize the patient for transport.dr jawed

Mental Illness

Some patients arrive at an emergency department for a complaint of mental illness. In many jurisdictions (including many U.S. states), patients who appear to be mentally ill and to present a danger to themselves or others may be brought against their will to an emergency department by law enforcement officers for psychiatric examination. The emergency department conducts medical clearance rather and treats acute behavioural disorders. From the emergency department, patients with significant mentally illness may be transferred to a psychiatric unit (in many cases involuntarily).

Asthma and COPD

Acute exacerbations of chronic respiratory diseases, mainly asthma and chronic obstructive pulmonary disease (COPD), are assessed as emergencies and treated with oxygen therapy, bronchodilators, steroids or theophylline, have an urgent chest X-ray and arterial blood gases and are referred for intensive care if necessary. Non invasive ventilation in the ED has reduced the requirement for intubation in many cases of severe exacerbations of COPD.

Special Facilities, Training, and Equipment

An ED requires different equipment and different approaches than most other hospital divisions. Patients frequently arrive with unstable conditions, and so must be treated quickly. They may be unconscious, and information such as their medical history, allergies, and blood type may be unavailable. ED staff are trained to work quickly and effectively even with minimal information.

ED staff must also interact efficiently with pre-hospital care providers such as EMTs, paramedics, and others who are occasionally based in an ED. The pre-hospital providers may use equipment unfamiliar to the average physician, but ED physicians must be expert in using (and safely removing) specialized equipment, since devices such as Military Anti-Shock Trousers ("MAST") and traction splints require special procedures. Among other reasons, given that they must be able to handle specialized equipment, physicians can now specialize in emergency medicine, and EDs employ many such specialists.

ED staff have much in common with ambulance and fire crews, combat medics, search and rescue teams, and disaster response teams. Often, joint training and practice drills are organized to improve the coordination of this complex response system. Busy EDs exchange a great deal of equipment with ambulance crews, and both must provide for replacing, returning, or reimbursing for costly items.

Cardiac arrest and major trauma are relatively common in EDs, so defibrillators, automatic ventilation and CPR machines, and bleeding control dressings are used heavily. Survival in such cases is greatly enhanced by shortening the wait for key interventions, and in recent years some of this specialized equipment has spread to pre-hospital settings. The best-known example is defibrillators, which spread first to ambulances, then in an automatic version to police cars, and most recently to public spaces such as airports, office buildings, hotels, and even shopping malls.

Because time is such an essential factor in emergency treatment, EDs typically have their own diagnostic equipment to avoid waiting for equipment installed elsewhere in the hospital. Nearly all have an X-ray room, and many now have full radiology facilities including CT scanners and ultrasonography equipment. Laboratory services may be handled on a priority basis by the hospital lab, or the ED may have its own "STAT Lab" for basic labs (blood counts, blood typing, toxicology screens, etc.) that must be returned very rapidly.

Non-emergency Use

Metrics applicable to the ED can be grouped into three main categories, volume, cycle time, and patient satisfaction. Volume metrics including arrivals per hour, percentage of ED beds occupied and age of patients are understood at a basic level at all hospitals as an indication for staffing requirements. Cycle time metrics are the mainstays of the evaluation and tracking of process efficiency and are less widespread since an active effort is needed to collect and analyze this data.

Patient satisfaction metrics, already commonly collected by physician groups and hospitals, are useful in demonstrating the impact of changes in patient perception of care over time. Since patient satisfaction metrics are derivative and subjective, they are less useful in primary process improvement.

In many Primary Care Trusts there may be out of hours doctor services sometimes known as Keydoc or something similar (varying by area) provided by volunteer General Practitioners.

Patients attending the ED for minor complaints do not contribute significantly to the overall workload of the department. (Despite the level of complaints in the general public and by health staff.) Studies, in Australia at least, have shown that improved after-hours GP access has no effect on ED workload or waiting times.

In the United States, and many other countries, hospitals are beginning to create areas in their emergency rooms for people with minor injuries. These are commonly referred as *fast track* or Minor Care units. These units are for people with non life-threatening injuries. The use of these units within a department have been shown to significantly improve the flow of patients through a department and to reduce waiting times. Urgent care clinics are another alternative, where patients can go to receive immediate care for non-life-threatening conditions.

Doctors in Training

Doctors in training provide a large portion of the medical care in emergency departments.

In the United States, they are called residents and are supervised by ABEM board certified attending physicians.

In the United Kingdom, many doctors rotate through the emergency department, such as during their second foundation year (F2), or as part of a rotational specialty training programme in General Practice or Emergency Medicine.

Emergency Departments in the Military

Emergency departments in the military benefit from the added support of enlisted personnel who are capable of performing any task they have been trained for, regardless of actual education obtained from civilian schooling. For example, in Naval hospitals, Hospital Corpsmen perform tasks that fall under the scope of practice of both doctors (i.e. sutures and incision and drainages) and nurses (i.e. medication administration and foley catheter insertion). Often, some civilian education and/or certification will be required such as an EMT certification, in case of the need to provide care outside of the base where the member is actually stationed.

Geriatric Intensive-care Unit

Geriatric intensive care unit is a special type of intensive care unit dedicated to management of critically ill elderly.

Geriatric intensive care unit's goal is to restore physiologic stability, prevent complications, maintain comfort and safety, and preserve pre-illness functional ability and quality of life (QOL) in older adults admitted to critical-care units.

Origin

Geriatric intensive care units appeared in response to the world's population aging. Managing Geriatrics diseases is not like managing adults or pediatrics diseases, especially if they are critically ill. Geriatric medicine was not included in the curricula of undergraduate or advanced medical training until recently, so not all critical care physicians were oriented by the pecularties of geriatric patients.

Despite the fact that geriatric patients constitute many of the critically ill patients, the training of critical care team still lacks the training on the geriatrics giants.

Critically ill older adult: a person, age 65 or older, who is currently experiencing or at risk for some form of physiologic instability or alteration warranting urgent or emergent, advanced nursing/medical interventions and monitoring.

- More than half (55.8%) of all ICU days are incurred by patients older than 65.
- Older adults are living longer, are more racially and ethnically diverse, often have multiple chronic conditions, and more than one-quarter report difficulty performing one or more activities of daily living (ADLs). These factors may affect both the course and outcome of critical illness.
- Once hospitalized for a life-threatening illness, older adults often:

1. Experience high ICU, hospital, and long-term crude mortality rates.
2. Are at risk for deterioration in functional ability and post-discharge institutional care.

- Older age is also a factor that may lead to:
  1. Physician bias in refusing ICU admission.
  2. The decision to withhold mechanical ventilation, surgery, or dialysis.
  3. An increased likelihood of an established resuscitation directive.
- Most critically ill older adults:
  1. Demonstrate resiliency.
  2. Report being satisfied with their QOL post-discharge.
  3. Would reaccept ICU care and mechanical ventilation if needed.
- Chronologic age alone is not an acceptable or accurate predictor of poor outcomes after critical illness.
- Factors that may influence an older adult's ability to survive a catastrophic illness include:
  1. Severity of illness
  2. Nature and extent of co-morbidities
  3. Diagnosis, reason for/duration of mechanical ventilation
  4. Complications length of ICU/hospital stay.

Goal

Goal is to restore physiologic stability, prevent complications, maintain comfort and safety, and preserve pre-illness functional ability and quality of life (QOL) in older adults admitted to critical-care units.

Distribution in the World

Geriatric intensive care units are starting to be disseminated and are currently present in Japan, USA, China, Egypt, India & Europe (France, Italy, Poland, Germany).

Practice Issues

Critical care practice by necessity is focused on the physiological parameters of the patients being served. Thus, the most important effort revolves around maintaining physiological function and restoring homeostasis for the person who is critically ill. However, when the urgent episode subsides, inappropriate practice guidelines and clinical approaches are often used in the care of older adults.

Older individuals have less physiological reserve than younger ones and, therefore, are more likely to have dire consequences following critical care events such as cardiac or respiratory arrest. Further, there are associated geriatric syndromes, medication issues and problems that can be prevented if they are anticipated. Sleep disorders are prevalent in the elderly. During a critical care episode, sleeping and waking cycles are disturbed. Because of the noise in an ICU, less sleep and more noise may trigger delirium. Improving critical care practice for the elderly requires attention to sleep deficits, which means appropriate rest and recovery time.

Altered Eating and Feeding Patterns are commoner in geriatric intensive care units. Tubes and other devices, which can impede the ability to obtain adequate nutrition, are common in an intensive care unit. While total parenteral nutrition lines can be inserted to provide calories, the pleasure of eating is lost, as is the sensory stimulation (i.e., smell, taste, texture) of the food, which might increase appetite.

Careful attention must be paid to weight loss in the elderly during the critical care episode. Because albumin levels may already be potentially compromised, the older individual will be at risk for pressure ulcers if their nutrition falls to critically low levels. Other reasons for impaired nutrition include mouth sores; dry, cracked mouths; or a lack of dentures. These issues may be overlooked in busy units.

Foley catheters are regularly inserted in patients in the intensive care unit to monitor fluid balance, this should be changed. urinary catheters are known to cause urinary tract infections, which are potentially lethal to the elderly. Thus, when possible, catheters should be avoided in the ICU. In addition, the use of incontinence undergarments should be avoided, given the propensity for skin irritation and breakdown.

The ICU environment has been linked to delirium in the elderly. Disorientation to time or place because of overstimulation, pain and metabolic imbalances frequently results in cognitive changes. Optimally, critical care nurses must obtain a baseline mental status on the older patient upon admission and follow the changes through the use of a standardized assessment instrument such as a Mini-Mental State Examination. Early detection and intervention can reduce the use of either physical or chemical restraints.

Elderly admitted to intensive care units need special management as regard pharmacotherapy. They can suffer from special cardiovascular diseases, severe infections as MRSA of systemic fungal infections. And may need special posoperative analgesia. Also elderly need assessment by special instruments to predict the prognosis of ICU patients older than 75 years.

Ethical Issues

Geriatrics critical care dictate many ethical issues which have been put into the focus of some researches & discussions. Also visiting hours in the geriatric ICU need special organisation different from other ICUs.

Not only do critical care units utilize up to a third of hospital expenditures and about 1% of GNP, the critically ill elderly consume a disproportionate amount of ICU resources. Outcome prediction models for very elderly critically ill patients have been proposed with age as one of numerous model variables; but such models have not been widely validated. Despite the burgeoning emphasis on evidence-based population approach to health care, there is insufficient research to guide the critical care clinician. There remains a modicum of subjectivity in crucial decisions that affect the elderly patient receiving intensive care.

Older age is also one of the factors that lead to a physician bias in refusing ICU admission. Many Critical care physicians generally consider their older patients' quality of life to be worse than do the patients, although other studies that have assessed the quality of live show no age-related differences among ICU survivors. Furthermore, physicians' estimations of patient quality of life significantly influence physicians' attitudes to futility of care issues, in contrast to patients' perceptions.

Threshold for life-sustaining treatment in the elderly will continue to be different among the ICUs. Clinical decisions will be subjected to many ethical, legal, and socioeconomic pressures. Personal and religious beliefs will inevitably influence societal expectations and clinician practices. Severity of illness has the biggest influence on outcome in a critical illness. Age alone is not a predictor of short-term or long-term outcome in the older patient who is critically ill. Critical illness in the elderly remains a fertile area for future research. Also some people tend to put a stigma on the geriatric intensive-care patient in community and in games.

Some studies suggest that patients who are perceived not to benefit from critical care are more often refused intensive care unit admission; refusal is associated with an increased risk of hospital death. During times of decreased critical bed availability, several factors, including age, illness severity, and medical diagnosis, are used to triage patients, although their relative importance is uncertain.

Some studies suggest the solution of subintensive care units. Which are now present in many places.

Training & Education Programs

Geriatric intensive care unit physicians are trained in geriatric medicine & critical care medicine. Some Universities & medical schools offer training sessions on Geritric critical care medicine. Some books focusing on older patients in the emergency department and critical care unit are available. And other online resources.

Geriatric intensive care unit nurses receive special training in critical care of elderly in their basic training, advanced and clinical training. Some Nursing school faculties are establishing research in Geriatric critical care nursing. And a Geriatric Critical Care Nursing Research (GCCNR) Group was established, the purpose of this group is to serve as a forum to share, query, and exchange ideas and strategies related to the research involving and benefiting older ICU patients.

Intensive-care Unit

An intensive care unit (ICU), critical care unit (CCU), intensive therapy unit or intensive treatment unit (ITU) is a specialized department used in many countries' hospitals that provides intensive care medicine. Many hospitals also have designated intensive care areas for certain specialities of medicine, as dictated by the needs and available resources of each hospital. The naming is not rigidly standardized.

History

In 1854, Florence Nightingale left for the Crimean War, where the necessity to separate seriously wounded soldiers from less-seriously wounded was observed. Nightingale reduced mortality from 40% to 2% on the battlefield, creating the concept of intensive care

In 1950, anesthesiologist Peter Safar established the concept of "Advanced Support of Life," keeping patients sedated and ventilated in an intensive care environment. Safar is considered the first intensivist.

In response to a polio epidemic (where many patients required constant ventilation and surveillance), Bjorn Ibsen established the first intensive care unit in Copenhagen in 1953. The first application of this idea in the United States was pioneered by Dr. William Mosenthal, a surgeon at the Dartmouth-Hitchcock Medical Centre. In the 1960s, the importance of cardiac arrhythmias as a source of morbidity and mortality in myocardial infarctions (heart attacks) was recognized. This led to the routine use of cardiac monitoring in ICUs, especially in the post-MI setting.

Types

Specialized types of ICUs include:

- Neonatal intensive-care unit (NICU)
- Special Care Nursery (SCN)
- Pediatric intensive-care unit (PICU)

- Psychiatric intensive-care unit (PICU)
- Coronary care unit (CCU) for heart disease
- Cardiac Surgery intensive-care unit (CSICU)
- Cardiovascular intensive-care unit (CVICU)
- Medical intensive-care unit (MICU)
- Medical Surgical intensive-care unit (MSICU)
- Surgical intensive-care unit (SICU)
- Overnight intensive recovery (OIR)
- Neuroscience/Neurotrauma intensive-care unit (NICU)
- Neurointensive-care unit (NICU)
- Burn intensive-care unit (BWICU)
- Trauma Intensive care Unit (TICU)
- Shock Trauma intensive-care unit (STICU)
- Trauma-Neuro Critical Care intensive-care unit (TNCC)
- Respiratory intensive-care unit (RICU)
- Geriatric intensive-care unit (GICU).

Equipment and Systems

Common equipment in an ICU includes mechanical ventilator to assist breathing through an endotracheal tube or a tracheotomy opening; cardiac monitors including telemetry, external pacemakers, and defibrillators; dialysis equipment for renal problems; equipment for the constant monitoring of bodily functions; a web of intravenous lines, feeding tubes, nasogastric tubes, suction pumps, drains and catheters; and a wide array of drugs to treat the main condition(s). Medically induced comas, analgesics, and induced sedation reduce pain and prevent secondary infections.

Quality of Care

Medicine suggests a relation between ICU volume and quality of care for mechanically ventilated patients. After adjustment for severity of illness, demographic variables, and characteristics of the ICUs (including staffing by intensivists), higher ICU volume was significantly associated with lower ICU and hospital mortality rates. Typically, patient to nurse ratio is what determines the care. A ratio of 2 patients to 1 nurse is recommended for a medical ICU. This is unlike the ratio of 4:1 or 5:1 ratio on the medical floors.

Staff

Medical staff typically includes intensivists with training in internal medicine, surgery, anesthesia, or emergency medicine. Many nurse practitioners and physician assistants with specialized training are also now part of the staff that provide continuity of care for patients. Staff typically includes specially trained critical care registered nurses, registered respiratory therapists, clinical pharmacists, nutritionists, physical therapists, certified nursing assistants, social workers etc.

Intensive Care Around the World

In the United Kingdom intensive care medicine is an extremely specialised area. In the United States up to 20% of hospital beds can be labelled as intensive care beds, whereas in the United Kingdom intensive care usually will comprise only up to 2% of total beds. This high disparity is attributed to patients in the UK who are admitted to an ICU tending to be only the most severely ill.

Intensive Care is an incredibly expensive healthcare service. In the United Kingdom the average cost of funding an intensive care unit is:

- £838 per bed per day for a Neonatal Intensive Care Unit
- £1,702 per bed per day for a Pediatric Intensive Care Unit
- £1,328 per bed per day for an Adult Intensive Care Unit.

ICU Quality and Management Tools

The intensive care unit (ICU) is one of the major components of the current health care system. The advances in supportive care and monitoring resulted in significant improvements in the care of surgical and clinical patients. Nowadays aggressive surgical therapies as well as transplantation are made safer by the monitoring in a closed environment, the surgical ICU, in the post-operative period. Moreover, the care and full recovery of many severely ill clinical patients as those with life-threatening infections occurs as a result of intensive care.

However, despite many significant advances in various fields as mechanical ventilation, renal replacement therapy, antimicrobial therapy and hemodynamic monitoring this increased knowledge and the wise use of such technology is not available for all patients. Shortage of ICU beds are an important issue, however even when ICU beds are available significant variability in treatment and in the adherence to evidence-based interventions do not occur.

Tools for ICU Quality Monitoring

Several measures of ICU performance have been proposed in the past 30 years. It is intuitive, and correct, to assume that ICU mortality may be a useful marker of quality. However, crude mortality rates does not take into consideration the singular aspects of each specific patient population that is treated in a certain geographic region, hospital or ICU. Therefore approaches looking for standardized mortality ratios that are adjusted for disease severity, comorbidities and other clinical aspects are often sought. Severity of illness is usually evaluated by scoring systems that integrates clinical, physiologic and demographic variables. Scoring systems are interesting tools to describe ICU populations and explain their different outcomes. The most frequently used are the APACHE II, SAPS II and MPM. However, newer scores as APACHE IV and SAPS III have been recently introduced in clinical practice. More than only using scoring systems, one should search for a high rate of adherence to clinically effective interventions. Adherence to interventions as deep venous thrombosis prophylaxis, reduction of ICU-acquired infections, adequate sedation regimens and decreasing and reporting serious adverse events are essential and have been accepted as benchmarking of quality.

The complex task of collecting and analyzing data on performance measures are made easier when clinical information systems are available. Although several clinical information systems focus on important aspects as computerized physician order entry systems and individual patient tracking information, few have attempted to gather clinical information generating full reports that provide a panorama of the ICU performance and detailed data on several domains as mortality, length of stay, severity of illness, clinical scores, nosocomial infections, adverse events and adherence to good clinical practice. Through implementing quality initiatives, increasing the quality of care and patient safety are major and feasible goals. Such systems (for example: Epimed Monitor) are available for clinical use and may facilitate the process of care on a daily basis and provide data for an in-depth analysis of ICU performance.

Neonatal Intensive-care Unit

A neonatal intensive care unit, usually shortened NICU (sometimes pronounced "Nickyou") and also called a newborn intensive care unit, intensive care nursery (ICN), and special care baby unit (SCBU [pronounced "Skiboo"], especially in Great Britain), or a humidicrib, is a unit of a hospital specializing in the care of ill or premature newborn infants. The NICU is distinct from a special care nursery (SCN) in providing a high level of intensive care to premature infants while the SCN provides specialized care for infants with less severe medical problems.

NICUs were developed in the 1950s and 1960s by pediatricians to provide better temperature support, isolation from infection risk, specialized feeding, and greater access to specialized equipment and resources. Infants are cared for in incubators or "open warmers."

Some low birth weight infants need respiratory support ranging from extra oxygen (by head hood or nasal cannula) to continuous positive airway pressure (CPAP) or mechanical ventilation. Public access is limited, and staff and visitors are required to take precautions to reduce transmission of infection. Nearly all children's hospitals have NICUs, but they can often be found in large general hospitals as well.

A NICU is typically directed by one or more neonatologists and staffed by nurses, nurse practitioners, Nursery Nurses, physician assistants, resident physicians, and respiratory therapists. Many other ancillary services are necessary for a top-level NICU. Other physicians, especially those with "organ-defined" specialties often assist in the care of these infants.

Equipment

Incubator

An *incubator* (or *open warmer* or *isolette*) is an apparatus used to maintain environmental conditions suitable for a neonate, (newborn baby). It is used in preterm births.

Possible functions of a neonatal incubator are:

- Oxygenation, through oxygen supplementation by head hood or nasal cannula, or even continuous positive airway pressure (CPAP) or mechanical ventilation. Infant respiratory distress syndrome is the leading cause of death in preterm infants, and the main treatments are CPAP, in addition to administering surfactant and stabilizing the blood sugar, blood salts, and blood pressure.
- Observation: Modern neonatal intensive care involves sophisticated measurement of temperature, respiration, cardiac function, oxygenation, and brain activity.
- Protection from cold temperature, infection, noise, drafts and excess handling: Incubators may be described as bassinets enclosed in plastic, with climate control equipment designed to keep them warm and limit their exposure to germs.
- Provision of nutrition, through intravenous catheters
- Administration of medications.
- Maintaining fluid balance by providing fluid and keeping a high air humidity to prevent a too great loss from skin and respiratory evaporation.

A *transport incubator* is an incubator and the most necessary neonatal instruments in a transportable format, and is used when a sick or premature baby is moved, e.g. from one hospital to another, as from a community hospital to a larger medical centre with a proper neonatal intensive care unit.

It usually has a miniature ventilator, cardio-respiratory monitor, IV pump, pulse oximeter, and oxygen supply built into its frame.

Early years

Doctors took an increasing role in childbirth from the eighteenth century onwards. However, the care of newborn babies, sick or well, remained largely in the hands of mothers and midwives. Some baby incubators, similar to those used for hatching chicks, were devised in the late nineteenth century. In the United States these were shown at commercial exhibitions, complete with babies inside, until 1943. It wasn't until after the Second World War that special care baby units (SCBUs) were established in many hospitals. In Britain, early SCBUs opened in Birmingham and Bristol. At Southmead Hospital, Bristol, initial opposition from obstetricians lessened after quadruplets born there in 1948 were successfully cared for in the new unit. More resources became available - the first unit had been set up with £100. Most early units had little equipment and relied on careful nursing and observation.

Incubators were expensive so the whole room often was kept warm instead. Cross-infection between babies was greatly feared. Strict nursing routines involved staff wearing gowns and masks, constant hand washing and minimal handling of babies. Parents were sometimes allowed to watch through the windows of the unit. Much was learned about feeding - frequent, tiny feeds seemed best - and breathing. Oxygen was given freely until the end of the 1950s, when it was shown that the high concentrations reached inside incubators caused some babies to go blind. Monitoring conditions in the incubator, and the baby itself, was to become a major area of research. Although incubators provided oxygen and warmth, science in the 1950s was limited and it was not until later that technology played a larger role in the decline of infant mortality. Even though the elimination of infectious disease was mostly responsible for decline in infant mortality, low birth weight infant mortality remained high. Yet, because of medical advances in neonatology, low birth weight infants today are surviving on average 15 years more than low weight infants born in the 1950s.

Increasing Technology

By the 1970s SCBUs were an established part of hospitals in the developed world. In Britain, some early units ran community programmes, sending experienced nurses to help care for premature babies at home. But increasingly technological monitoring and therapy meant special care for babies became hospital-based. By the 1980s, over 90% of births took place in hospital anyway. The emergency dash from home to SCBU with baby in a transport incubator had become a thing of the past, though transport incubators were still needed. Specialist equipment and expertise were not available at every hospital, and strong arguments were made for large, centralised SCBUs. On the downside was the long travelling time for frail babies and for parents. A 1979 study showed that 20% of babies in SCBUs for up to a week were never visited by either parent. Centralised or not, by the 1980s few questioned the role of SCBUs in saving babies. Around 80% of babies born weighing under 1.5 kg now survived, compared to around 40% in the 1960s. From 1982 in Britain pediatricians could train and qualify in the sub-specialty of neonatal medicine.

Not only careful nursing, but also new techniques and instruments now played a major role. As in adult intensive care units, the use of monitoring and life support systems became routine. These needed special modification for small babies, whose bodies were tiny and often immature. Adult ventilators, for example, could damage babies lungs and gentler techniques with smaller pressure changes were devised. The many tubes and sensors used for monitoring the baby's condition, blood sampling and artificial feeding made some babies scarcely visible beneath the technology.

Furthermore, by 1975, over 18% of newborn babies in Britain were being admitted to SCBUs. Some hospitals admitted all babies delivered by Caesarian section, or under 2500g in weight. The fact that these babies missed early close contact with their mothers was a growing concern. As in other area of medicine, the 1980s saw questions being raised about the human, and the economic costs of too much technology. Admission policies gradually changed. In addition, treating low birth weight infants is expensive, especially when there are much cheaper ways of ensuring healthy babies. The key is prevention. Money can be spent on programs educating mothers on staying healthy during their pregnancy. One program (one that encourages women to stop smoking) is one third the price of neonatal intensive care and has been proven to work. During this program, a significant number of women often quit.

Changing Priorities

SCBUs now concentrate on treating very small, premature, or otherwise sick babies. Some of these babies are from higher-order multiple births, but most are still single babies born too early. Premature labour, and how to prevent it, remains a perplexing problem for doctors. Even though medical advancements allow doctors to save low birth weight babies, it is almost invariably better to delay such births.

Over the last 10 years or so, SCBUs have become much more 'parent friendly', encouraging maximum involvement with the babies. Routine gowns and masks have gone and parents are encouraged to help with care as much as possible. Cuddling, and skin-to-skin contact, also known as Kangaroo care, are seen as beneficial for all but the frailest (very tiny babies are exhausted by the stimulus of being handled, or larger critically ill infants). Less stressful ways of delivering high-technology medicine to tiny patients have been devised - stick-on sensors to measure blood oxygen levels through the skin, for example, and ways of reducing the amount of blood taken for tests.

Some major problems of the SCBU have almost disappeared. Exchange transfusions, in which all the blood is removed and replaced, little by little, are rare now. Rhesus incompatibility (a difference in blood groups) between mother and baby is largely preventable. Breathing difficulties and brain hemorrhage still claim many infant lives and are the focus of many current research projects.

The long term outlook for premature babies saved by SCBUs has always been a concern. From the early years, it was reported that a higher proportion than normal grew up with disabilities, including cerebral palsy and learning difficulties. Now that treatments are available for many of the problems faced by tiny or immature babies in the first weeks of life, long-term follow-up, and minimising long-term disability, are major research areas.

Besides prematurity and extreme low birth weight, common diseases cared for in a NICU include perinatal asphyxia, extreme cases of preeclampsia/eclampsia, major birth defects, sepsis, neonatal jaundice, and respiratory distress syndrome due to immaturity of the lungs. The leading cause of death in NICUs is generally necrotizing enterocolitis. Complications of extreme prematurity may include intracranial hemorrhage, chronic bronchopulmonary dysplasia, or retinopathy of prematurity. An infant may spend a day of observation in a NICU or may spend many months there. Overall survival rates, for all gestational ages lumped together, are roughly 70%.

Neonatology and NICUs have greatly increased the survival of very low birth weight and extremely premature infants. In the era before NICUs, infants of birth weight less than 1400 grams (3 lb, usually about 30 weeks gestation) rarely survived. Today, infants of 500 grams at 26 weeks have a fair chance of survival.

The NICU environment provides challenges as well as benefits. Stressors for the infants can include continual light, a high level of noise, separation from their mothers, reduced physical contact, painful procedures, and interference with the opportunity to breastfeed. A NICU can be stressful for the staff as well. A special aspect of NICU stress for both parents and staff is that infants may survive, but with damage to the brain or eyes.

NICU rotations are essential aspects of pediatric and obstetric residency programs, but NICU experience is encouraged by other specialty residencies, such as family practice, surgery, Pharmacy, and emergency medicine.

2

Nursing

Nursing is a healthcare profession focused on the care of individuals, families, and communities so they may attain, maintain, or recover optimal health and quality of life from birth to death.

Nurses work in a large variety of specialties where they work independently and as part of a team to assess, plan, implement and evaluate care.

History of Nursing

Nursing comes in various forms in every culture, although the definition of the term and the practice of nursing has being known as a wet nurse and the latter being known as a *dry nurse*. In the 15th century, this developed into the idea of looking after or advising another, not necessarily meaning a woman looking after a child. Nursing has continued to develop in this latter sense, although the idea of nourishing in the broadest sense refers in modern nursing to promoting quality of life.

Prior to the foundation of modern nursing, nuns and the military often provided nursing-like services. The religious and military roots of modern nursing remain in evidence today in many countries, for example in the United Kingdom, senior female nurses are known as "sisters". It was during time of war that a significant development in nursing history arose when English nurse Florence Nightingale, working to improve conditions of soldiers in the Crimean War, laid the foundation stone of professional nursing with the principles summarised in the book

Notes on Nursing. Other important nurses in the development of the profession include: Mary Seacole, who also worked as a nurse in the Crimea; Agnes Elizabeth Jones and Linda Richards, who established quality nursing schools in the USA and Japan, and Linda Richards who was officially America's first trained nurse, graduating in 1873 from the *New England Hospital for Women and Children* in Boston.

New Zealand was the first country to regulate nurses nationally, with adoption of the Nurses Registration Act on the 12th of September, 1901. Ellen Dougherty was the first registered nurse. North Carolina was the first state in the United States to pass a nursing licensure law in 1903.

Nurses have experienced difficulty with the hierarchy in medicine that has resulted in an impression that nurses primary purpose is to follow the direction of medics. This tendency is certainly not observed in Nightingale's *Notes on Nursing*, where the doctors are mentioned relatively infrequently and often in critical tones, particularly relating to bedside manner.

The modern era has seen the development of nursing degrees and nursing has numerous journals to broaden the knowledge base of the profession. Nurses are often in key management roles within health services and hold research posts at universities.

Nursing as a Profession

The authority for the practice of nursing is based upon a social contract that delineates professional rights and responsibilities as well as mechanisms for public accountability. In almost all countries, nursing practice is defined and governed by law, and entrance to the profession is regulated at national or state level.

The aim of the nursing community worldwide is for its professionals to ensure quality care for all, while maintaining their credentials, code of ethics, standards, and competencies, and continuing their education. There are a number of educational paths to becoming a professional nurse, which vary greatly worldwide, but all involve extensive study of nursing theory and practice and training in clinical skills. Nurses care for individuals who are healthy and ill, of all ages 99 and cultural backgrounds, and who have physical, emotional, psychological, intellectual, social, and spiritual needs. The profession combines physical science, social science, nursing theory, and technology in caring for those individuals.

In order to work in the nursing profession, all nurses hold one or more credentials depending on their scope of practice and education. A Licensed practical nurse (LPN) (also referred to as a Licensed vocational nurse, Registered practical nurse, Enrolled nurse, and State enrolled nurse) works under a Registered nurse. A Registered nurse (RN) provides scientific, psychological, and technological knowledge in the care of patients and families in many health care settings. Registered nurses may also earn additional credentials or degrees enabling them to work under different titles.

Nurses may follow their personal and professional interests by working with any group of people, in any setting, at any time. Some nurses follow the traditional role of working in a hospital setting.

Nursing Practice

Nursing practice is primarily the caring relationship between the nurse and the person in their care. In providing nursing care, nurses are implementing the nursing care plan, which is based on a nursing assessment.

Nursing Theory and Process

In general terms, the nursing process is the method used to assess and diagnose needs, plan and implement interventions, and evaluate the outcomes of the care provided. Like other disciplines, the profession has developed different theories derived from sometimes diverse philosophical beliefs and paradigms or worldviews to help nurses direct their activities to accomplish specific goals. Currently, two paradigms exist in nursing, the totality paradigm and the simultaneity paradigm.

Practice Settings

Nurses practice in a wide range of settings, from hospitals to visiting people in their homes and caring for them in schools to research in pharmaceutical companies. Nurses work in occupational health settings (also called industrial health settings), free-standing clinics and physician offices, nurse-run clinics, long-term care facilities and camps. They also work on cruise ships and in military service. Nurses act as advisers and consultants to the health care and insurance industries. Some are attorneys and others work with attorneys as legal nurse consultants, reviewing patient records to assure that adequate care was provided and testifying in court. Nurses can work on a temporary basis, which involves doing shifts without a contact in a variety of settings, sometimes known as *per diem* nursing, agency nursing or travel nursing. Nurses work as researchers in laboratories, universities and research institutions.

Work Environment

Internationally, there is a serious shortage of nurses. One reason for this shortage is due to the work environment in which nurses practice. In a recent review of the empirical human factors and ergonomic literature specific to nursing performance, nurses were found to work in generally poor environmental conditions. DeLucia, Ott, & Palmieri (2009) concluded, "the profession of nursing as a whole is overloaded because there is a nursing shortage. Individual nurses are overloaded. They are overloaded by the number of patients they oversee. They are overloaded by the number of tasks they perform. They work under cognitive overload, engaging in multitasking and encountering frequent interruptions. They work under perceptual overload due to medical devices that do not meet perceptual requirements (Morrow et al., 2005), insufficient lighting, illegible handwriting, and poor labeling designs. They work under physical overload due to long work hours and patient handling demands which leads to a high incidence of MSDs. In short, the nursing work system often exceeds the limits and capabilities of human performance. HF/E research should be conducted to determine how these overloads can be reduced and how the limits and capabilities of performance can be accommodated. Ironically, the literature shows that there are studies to determine whether nurses can effectively perform tasks ordinarily performed by physicians. Results indicate that nurses can perform such tasks effectively. Nevertheless, already overloaded nurses should not be given more tasks to perform. When reducing the overload, it should be kept in mind that underloads also can be detrimental to performance (Mackworth, 1948). Considering both overloads and underloads are important to consider for improving performance."

Regulation of Practice

The practice of nursing is governed by laws that define a scope of practice, generally mandated by the legislature of the political division within which the nurse practices. Nurses are held legally responsible and accountable for their practice. The standard of care is that of the "prudent nurse."

Nursing Specialties

Nursin~ ·~ the most diverse of all healthcare professions. Nurses practice in ide range of settings but generally nursing is divided depending on the needs of the person being nursed.

The major divisions are:-

- the nursing of people with mental health problems - Psychiatric and mental health nursing
- the nursing of people with learning or developmental disabilities - Learning disability nursing (UK)
- the nursing of children - Pediatric nursing.
- the nursing of older adults - Geriatric nursing
- the nursing of people in acute care and long term care institutional settings.
- the nursing of people in their own homes - Home health nursing (US), District nursing and Health visiting (UK).

There are also specialist areas such as cardiac nursing, orthopedic nursing, palliative care, perioperative nursing and oncology nursing, or the specialization to cancer.

Nursing Unit

A nursing unit is an area in a hospital or other health care delivery setting where patients with similar needs are grouped to facilitate the delivery of care by health care professionals trained in that specialty. Typically a nurse manager or matron is in charge of the unit.

Types of Nursing Units

Inpatient Units

- Bone marrow transplant
- Burn unit
- Geriatrics
- Hematology/Oncology
- Labor and Delivery
- Cardiology
- Medical/Surgical (frequently abbreviated as "Med/Surg")
- Medicine
- Mother/Baby
- Neurology
- Neurosurgery
- Neuropsychiatric
- Oncology
- Organ transplant
- Orthopaedics
- Otolaryngology
- Pediatrics
- Psychiatry
- Rehabilitation
- Surgery
- Telemetry
- Urology.

Outpatient clinics

- Burn treatment
- Diabetes

- Disabilities and developmental disorders
- Chemical dependency
- Dermatology
- Diagnostic Radiology
- Emergency treatment
- Medicine
- Neurology
- Neurosurgery
- Oncology
- Oral surgery
- Orthopaedics
- Otolaryngology
- Pediatrics
- Psychiatry
- Radiation oncology
- Renal dialysis
- Rheumatology
- Surgical
- Urology.

Intensive care units

- Cardiovascular intensive care unit (CCU)
- Medical intensive care unit (MICU)
- Neonatal intensive care unit (NICU)
- Pediatric intensive care unit (PICU)
- Step-down care units
- Surgical intensive care unit (SICU).

Surgical units

- Ambulatory surgery
- Main operating room
- Post-anesthesia care unit (PACU).

On-call room

An on-call room is a room in a hospital with either a couch or a bunkbed intended for staff to rest in while they are on-call or due to be.

In the European Community, the 2003 extension of the working time directive to junior doctors and the ruling that on-call time counts as working hours has resulted in the introduction of shift working for hospital medical staff, thereby eliminating the requirements for on-call rooms.

Physical therapy

Physical therapy (also physiotherapy) is a health care profession that provides treatment to individuals to develop, maintain and restore maximum movement and function throughout life. This includes providing treatment in circumstances where movement and function are threatened by aging, injury, disease or environmental factors.

Physical therapy is concerned with identifying and maximizing quality of life and movement potential within the spheres of promotion, prevention, treatment/intervention, habilitation and rehabilitation. This encompasses physical, psychological, emotional, and social well being. It involves the interaction between physical therapist (PT), patients/clients, other health professionals, families, care givers, and communities in a process where movement potential is assessed and goals are agreed upon, using knowledge and skills unique to physical therapists. Physical therapy is performed by either a physical therapist (PT) or an assistant (PTA) acting under their direction.

PTs use an individual's history and physical examination to arrive at a diagnosis and establish a management plan and, when necessary, incorporate the results of laboratory and imaging studies. Electrodiagnostic testing (e.g., electromyograms and nerve conduction velocity testing) may also be of assistance.

Physical therapy has many specialties including cardiopulmonary, geriatrics, neurologic, orthopaedic and pediatrics, to name some of the more common areas. PTs practice in many settings, such as outpatient clinics or offices, inpatient rehabilitation facilities, skilled nursing facilities, extended care facilities, private homes, education and research centres, schools, hospices, industrial workplaces or other occupational environments, fitness centres and sports training facilities.

Education qualifications vary greatly by country. The span of education ranges from some countries having little formal education to others requiring masters or doctoral degrees.

History

Physicians like Hippocrates and later Galenus are believed to have been the first practitioners of physical therapy, advocating massage, manual therapy techniques and hydrotherapy to treat people in 460 B.C. After the development of orthopedics in the eighteenth century, machines like the Gymnasticon were developed to treat gout and similar diseases by systematic exercise of the joints, similar to later developments in physical therapy.

The earliest documented origins of actual physical therapy as a professional group date back to Per Henrik Ling "Father of Swedish Gymnastics" who founded the Royal Central Institute of Gymnastics (RCIG) in 813 for massage, manipulation, and exercise. The Swedish word for physical therapist is "sjukgymnast" = "sick-gymnast." In 1887, PTs were given official registration by Sweden's National Board of Health and Welfare.

Other countries soon followed. In 1894 four nurses in Great Britain formed the Chartered Society of Physiotherapy. The School of Physiotherapy at the University of Otago in New Zealand in 1913, and the United States' 1914 Reed College in Portland, Oregon, which graduated "reconstruction aides."

Research catalyzed the physical therapy movement. The first physical therapy research was published in the United States in March 1921 in *The PT Review*. In the same year, Mary McMillan organized the Physical Therapy Association (now called the American Physical Therapy Association (APTA). In 1924, the Georgia Warm Springs Foundation promoted the field by touting physical therapy as a treatment for polio.

Treatment through the 1940s primarily consisted of exercise, massage, and traction. Manipulative procedures to the spine and extremity joints began to be practiced, especially in the British Commonwealth countries, in the early 1950s. Later that decade, physical therapists started to move beyond hospital based practice, to outpatient orthopedic clinics, public schools, college/universities, geriatric settings (skilled nursing facilities), rehabilitation centres, hospitals, and medical centres.

Specialization for physical therapy in the U.S. occurred in 1974, with the Orthopaedic Section of the APTA being formed for those physical therapists specializing in orthopaedics. In the same year, the International Federation of Orthopaedic Manipulative Therapy was formed, which has played an important role in advancing manual therapy worldwide ever since.

Education

World Confederation of Physical Therapy (WCPT) recognises there is considerable diversity in the social, economic, cultural, and political environments in which physical therapist education is conducted throughout the world. WCPT recommends physical therapist entry-level educational programs be based on university or university-level studies, of a minimum of four years, independently validated and accredited as being at a standard that accords graduates full statutory and professional recognition. WCPT acknowledges there is innovation and variation in program delivery and in entry-level qualifications, including first university degrees (Bachelors/Baccalaureate/Licensed or equivalent), Masters and Doctorate entry qualifications. What is expected is that any program should deliver a curriculum that will enable physical therapists to attain the knowledge, skills, and attributes described in these guidelines. Professional education prepares physical therapists to be autonomous practitioners in collaboration with other members of the health care team.

Physical therapist entry-level educational programs integrate theory, evidence and practice along a continuum of learning. This begins with admission to an accredited physical therapy program and ending with retirement from active practice.

202 of 211 accredited physical therapy programs in the US are accredited at the doctoral level.

Specialty areas

Because the body of knowledge of physical therapy is quite large, some PTs specialize in a specific clinical area. While there are many different types of physical therapy, the American Board of Physical Therapy Specialties list seven specialist certifications, including Sports Physical Therapy and Clinical Electrophysiology. Worldwide the six most common specialty areas in physical therapy are:

Cardiopulmonary

Cardiovascular and pulmonary rehabilitation physical therapists treat a wide variety of individuals with cardiopulmonary disorders or those who have had cardiac or pulmonary surgery. Primary goals of this specialty include increasing endurance and functional independence. Manual therapy is used in this field to assist in clearing lung secretions experienced with cystic fibrosis. Disorders, including heart attacks, post coronary bypass surgery, chronic obstructive pulmonary disease, and pulmonary fibrosis, treatments can benefit from cardiovascular and pulmonary specialized physical therapists.

Geriatric

Geriatric physical therapy covers a wide area of issues concerning people as they go through normal adult aging but is usually focused on the older adult. There are many conditions that affect many people as they grow older and include but are not limited to the following: arthritis, osteoporosis, cancer, Alzheimer's disease, hip and joint replacement, balance disorders, incontinence, etc.

Geriatric physical therapy helps those affected by such problems in developing a specialized program to help restore mobility, reduce pain, and increase fitness levels.

Neurological

Neurological physical therapy is a discipline focused on working with individuals who have a neurological disorder or disease. These include Alzheimer's disease, Charcot-Marie-Tooth disease (CMT), ALS, brain injury, cerebral palsy, multiple sclerosis,

Parkinson's disease, spinal cord injury, and stroke. Common impairments associated with neurologic conditions include impairments of vision, balance, ambulation, activities of daily living, movement, speech and loss of functional independence.

Orthopaedic

Orthopaedic physical therapists diagnose, manage, and treat disorders and injuries of the musculoskeletal system including rehabilitation after orthopaedic surgery. This specialty of physical therapy is most often found in the out-patient clinical setting.

Orthopaedic therapists are trained in the treatment of post-operative orthopaedic procedures, fractures, acute sports injuries, arthritis, sprains, strains, back and neck pain, spinal conditions and amputations.

Joint and spine mobilization/manipulation, therapeutic exercise, neuromuscular reeducation, hot/cold packs, and electrical muscle stimulation (e.g., cryotherapy, iontophoresis, electrotherapy) are modalities often used to expedite recovery in the orthopaedic setting. Additionally, an emerging adjunct to diagnosis and treatment is the use of sonography for diagnosis and to guide treatments such as muscle retraining. Those who have suffered injury or disease affecting the muscles, bones, ligaments, or tendons of the body will benefit from assessment by a physical therapist specialized in orthopaedics.

Pediatric

Pediatric physical therapy assists in early detection of health problems and uses a wide variety of modalities to treat disorders in the pediatric population. These therapists are specialized in the diagnosis, treatment, and management of infants, children, and adolescents with a variety of congenital, developmental, neuromuscular, skeletal, or acquired disorders/diseases.

Treatments focus on improving gross and fine motor skills, balance and coordination, strength and endurance as well as cognitive and sensory processing/integration. Children with developmental delays, cerebral palsy, spina bifida, or torticollis, may be treated by pediatric physical therapists.

Integumentary

Integumentary (treatment of conditions involving the skin and related organs). Common conditions managed include wounds and burns. Physical therapists utilize surgical instruments, mechanical lavage, dressings and topical agents to debride necrotic tissue and promote tissue healing. Other commonly used interventions include exercise, edema control, splinting, and compression garments.

Occupational Therapy

Occupational therapy, often abbreviated as "OT", promotes health by enabling people to perform meaningful and purposeful occupations. These include (but are not limited to) work, leisure, self care, domestic and community activities. Occupational therapists work with individuals, families, groups and communities to facilitate health and well-being through engagement or re-engagement in occupation. Occupational therapists are becoming increasingly involved in addressing the impact of social, political and environmental factors that contribute to exclusion and occupational deprivation.

The World Federation of Occupational Therapists provides the following definition of Occupational Therapy: "Occupational therapy is as a profession concerned with promoting health and well being through occupation. The primary goal of occupational therapy is to enable people to participate in the activities of everyday life. Occupational therapists achieve this outcome by enabling people to do things that will enhance their ability to participate or by modifying the environment to better support participation."

Occupational therapists use careful analysis of physical, environmental, psychosocial, mental, spiritual, political and cultural factors to identify barriers to occupation. Occupational therapy draws from the fields of medicine, psychology, sociology, anthropology, ethnography, architecture and many other disciplines in developing its knowledge base. A new discipline of occupational science has been developed to enhance the evidence base of the profession.

History of Occupational Therapy

The earliest evidence of using occupations as a therapeutic modality can be found in ancient times. One-hundred years before the birth of Christ, Greek physician Asclepiades initiated humane treatment of patients with mental illness via the use of therapeutic baths, massage, exercise, and music. Later, the Roman Celsus prescribed music, travel, conversation and exercise to his patients. Unfortunately, by medieval times, the concept of humane treatment of people considered to be insane was rare, if not nonexistent.

In eighteenth century Europe, revolutionaries such as Philippe Pinel and Johann Christian Reil reformed the hospital system. Instead of the use of metal chains and restraint, their institutions utilized rigorous work and leisure activities in the late 1700s. Although it was thriving abroad, interest in the reform movement waxed and waned in the United States throughout the nineteenth century. At the turn of the 20th century, as physicians became increasingly interested in chronic disease, enthusiasm for the reform of the mental healthcare system was revived in the states. Work therapy found its way to America.

The health profession of occupational therapy as we know it was conceived in the early 1910s. Focus was on promoting health in "invalids." Early professionals merged highly valued ideals, such as having a strong work ethic and the importance of crafting with one's own hands, with scientific and medical principles. Early adversaries viewed wood carving and crafting by ill patients trivial.

The emergence of occupational therapy challenged the views of mainstream scientific medicine. Instead of focusing on purely physical etiologies, they argued that a complex combination of social, economic, and biological reasons cause dysfunction. Principles and techniques were borrowed from many disciplines—including but not limited to nursing, psychiatry, rehabilitation, self-help, orthopedics, and social work—to enrich the profession's scope. Between 1900 and 1930, the founders defined the realm of practice and developed theories of practice. In a short 20-year span, they successfully convinced the public and medical world of the value of occupational therapy and established standards for the profession. A substantial lack of primary sources of information has left today's occupational therapists with many questions concerning the founders of the field. Information is collected from early training institutions and hospitals, professional writings of practitioners, World War I records from government agencies, newspaper articles, and personal testimonials.

One of the most notable figures in the infancy of occupational therapy was Eleanor Clark Slagle. Slagle was part of the generation of women who challenged women's "rightful" place as a volunteer and strived for females to have a place in the professional world. At age forty, she was trained in curative occupations and recreations at the Chicago School of Civics and Philanthropy and later took a position at Hull House, where crafts were used to promote mental health.

It is speculated that Slagle's interest in healthcare stemmed from her personal life, as her father, brother, and nephew all suffered from various disabilities. Seeing the daily struggles of people with disabilities and illnesses may have sparked Slagle to enroll in the Chicago School in 1911. In 1912, renowned psychiatrist Adolph Meyer appointed Slagle to direct a new department of occupational therapy at John Hopkins Hospital. There, she learned habit training—a method of re-educating patients on decent habits of living via substituting healthful habits for bad habits.

Another psychiatrist, William Rush Dunton, Jr., worked diligently to raise the status of psychiatry in medicine in the first decades of the 20th century. He viewed occupational therapy as complementary to psychiatry, as it had the promise of meshing humanitarian values with science. Dunton became interested in the work of European moral therapy advocates. He accepted a position at the Sheppard Asylum, where it was standard practice in the early 1900s for patients to participate in activities such as bowling, gymnastics, art, etc. Dunton and his contemporaries called for the development of a theory to underlie the treatment known as "moral therapy" and "diversional occupation," among other names. He called for therapists to devise outcome measures so that the neophyte profession would be given the attention and respect he felt it deserved.

Another important figure in the early days of occupational therapy was Susan Tracy, a nurse by trade, who organized activity-oriented classes for nurses at the Adams Nervine Asylum. In 1910, she published a textbook that was widely used for over 30 years. She is credited with expanding the realm of occupational therapy from psychiatric institutions to the homes of patients, which is an important setting in which today's occupational therapists work. Upon breaking ties with the asylum, she set up her own institution, entitled the Experiment Station for the Study of Invalid Occupations. This training centre educated nurses so they could gain control over their practice and not default to being dominated by physicians. By practicing privately in patients' homes, this batch of occupational therapists expanded the domain of occupational therapy and began using OT to treat physical ailments as well as mental illness.

Herbert J. Hall was a physician with a strong work ethic and practical vision. He believed we could retract social ills by adapting the arts and crafts movement for medical purposes. A graduate of Harvard Medical School, he advised the government on wartime standards for occupational therapy during WWI. He introduced the concept of grading activities—now a hallmark of occupational therapy—to avoid exacerbating patient's frustration and fatigue.

George Edward Barton, although trained as an architect, was instrumental in the organization of occupational therapy as a profession. A man of many talents and broad interests, he had friends of varied backgrounds. (Barton was the librettist of the first American opera produced at the Metropolitan Opera House in New York.) Barton knew from his own personal experience the effects illness could take on the body and spirit. He was diagnosed with tuberculosis in 1901. Later, while working as the principal architect of the Myron Stratton Home (Colorado Springs, Colorado) Barton contracted frostbite, which became gangrene. He subsequently had a partial amputation, and was also partially paralyzed on his left side. He went to Clifton Springs, New York, to recuperate. In addition to his physical weakness, he suffered from emotional depression. After intensive self-administered occupational therapy, his ailments were "cured", if not completely, at least to the point where he was again able to contribute to society. He opened Consolation House in 1914, as the name suggests, as a sanctuary for people with physical disabilities. He played an integral part in forming the first national society by gathering together like-minded thinkers who became the profession's leaders.

The first meeting of the National Society for the Promotion of Occupational Therapy was held in March 1917. Barton, Secretary Isabel Gladwin Newton (whom he later married), Eleanor Clark Slagle, William Rush Dunton Jr., Thomas B. Kinder, and Susan Cox Johnson were the only six in attendance. By the fall of 1919, at the third meeting, 300 attendees participated. In 1921, the name of the organization was changed to the American Occupational Therapy Association, and the first professional journal, the Archives of Occupational Therapy, began publication.

World War I forced the new profession to clarify its role in the medical domain and to standardize training and practice. In addition to clarifying its public image, OT also established clinics, workshops, and training schools nationwide. Due to the overwhelming number of wartime injuries, "reconstruction aides" (an umbrella term for physical therapists and occupational therapists) were recruited by the Surgeon General. Between 1917 and 1920, nearly 148,000 wounded men were placed in hospitals upon their return to the states. This number does not account for those wounded abroad. The success of the reconstruction aides, largely made up of women trying to "do their bit" to help with the war effort, was a great accomplishment. Post-war, however, there was a struggle to keep people in the profession. Emphasis was shifted from the altruistic war-time mentality to the financial, professional, and personal satisfaction that comes with being a therapist. To make the profession more appealing, practice was standardized, as was the curriculum. Entry and exit criterion were established, and AOTA advocated for steady employment, decent wages, and fair working conditions. Via these methods, occupational therapy sought and obtained medical legitimacy in the 1920s. By the time Slagle retired from the profession in 1937, the profession's medical identity was well on its way to being established.

Evolution of the Philosophy of Occupational Therapy

The philosophy of occupational therapy has evolved over the history of the profession. The philosophy articulated by the founders that have owed much to the ideals of romanticism, pragmatism and humanism which are collectively considered the fundamental ideologies of the past century.

William Rush Dunton, the creator of the National Society for the Promotion of Occupational Therapy, now the American Occupational Therapy Association, sought to promote the ideas that occupation is a basic human need, and that occupation was therapeutic. From his statements, came some of the basic assumptions of occupational therapy, which include:

- Occupation has an effect on health and well-being.
- Occupation creates structure and organizes time.
- Occupation brings meaning to life, culturally and personally.
- Occupations are individual. People value different occupations.

These have been elaborated over time to form the values which underpin the Codes of Ethics issued by each national association. However, the relevance of occupation to health and well-being remains the central theme. Influenced by criticism from medicine and the multitude of physical disabilities resulting from World War II , occupational therapy adopted a more reductionistic philosophy for a time. While this approach lead to developments in technical knowledge about occupational performance, clinicians became increasingly disillusioned and re-considered these beliefs. As a result, client centeredness and occupation are re-emerging as dominant themes in the profession, perhaps indicating growing maturity and self confidence. Over the past century, the underlying philosophy of occupational therapy has evolved from being a diversion from illness, to treatment, to enablement through meaningful occupation. This became evident through the development and widespread adoption of the Canadian Model of Occupational Performance. The two most commonly mentioned values are that occupation is essential for health and the concept of holism. However, there have been some dissenting voices. Mocellin in particular advocated abandoning the notion of health through occupation as obsolete in the modern world and questioned the appropriateness of advocating holism when practice rarely supports it. The values formulated by the American Association of Occupational Therapists have also been critiqued as being therapist centred and not reflecting the modern reality of multicultural practice.

Central to the philosophy of occupational therapy is the concept of occupational performance. In considering occupational performance the therapist must consider the many factors which comprise overall performance. This concept is made more tangible using models such as the person-environment-occupation model proposed by Law et al. (1996). This approach highlights the importance of satisfactions in one's occupations, broadening the aim of occupational therapy beyond the mere completion of tasks to the holistic achievement of personal wellbeing.

In recent times occupational therapists have challenged themselves to think more broadly about the potential scope of the profession, and expanded it to include working with groups experiencing occupational deprivation which stems from sources other than disability. Examples of new and emerging practice areas would include therapists working with refugees, and with people experiencing homelessness.

Occupation, Occupational form and Performance

Occupation

Occupation is the dynamic relationship between the occupational form and occupational performance.

Many people see the term occupation as a job one does. However, the meaning of occupation is seen in a much wider context by an Occupational Therapist. A human being can be engaged in a wide range of occupations: leisure, selfcare or educational activities are just a few examples of occupation.

Occupational Form

Wu and Lin (2010) stated that the occupational form was the

"...objective pre-existing structure or environmental context that elicits or guides subsequent human performance". The occupational form consists of objective features. These may include materials, human context and socio-cultural dimensions.

Occupational Performance

Occupational performance is the active voluntary human doing of the occupational form.

Occupational Therapy Process

An Occupational Therapist works systematically through a sequence of actions known as the occupational therapy process. There are several versions of this process as described by numerous writers. Creek (2003) has sought to provide a comprehensive version based on extensive research. This version has 11 stages, which for the experienced therapist may not be linear in nature. The stages are:

- Referral
- Information gathering
- Initial assessment
- Needs identification/problem formation
- Goal setting
- Action planning
- Action
- Ongoing assessment and revision of action
- Outcome and outcome measurement
- End of intervention or discharge
- Review.

Fearing, Law and Clark (1997) suggested a 7 stage process which includes:

- identifying of occupational performance issues
- choosing a theoretical frame of reference
- assessing factors contributing the identified occupational performance issue(s)

- considering the strengths and resources of both client and therapist
- negotiating targeted outcomes and developing an action plan
- implementing the plan through occupation
- evaluating outcomes.

A central element of this process model is the focus on identifying both client and therapists strengths and resources prior to beginning to develop the outcomes and action plan.

Areas of Practice in Occupational Therapy

The role of Occupational Therapy allows OT's to work in many different settings, work with many different populations and acquire many different specialties. This broad spectrum of practice lends itself to difficulty categorizing the areas of practice that exist, especially considering the many countries and different healthcare systems. In this section, the categorization from the American Occupational Therapy Association is used. However, there are other ways to categorize areas of practice in OT, such as physical, mental, and community practice (AOTA, 2009). These divisions occur when the setting is defined by the population it serves. For example, acute physical or mental health settings (e.g.: hospitals), sub-acute settings (e.g.: aged care facilities), outpatient clinics and community settings.

In each area of practice below, an OT can work with different populations, diagnosis, specialities, and in different settings.

Physical Health

Pediatrics - Schools, Community, inpatient hospital based child OT: Often, children need OT services for the same reasons an adult needs OT services. However, OTs approach intervention in a different way with children. OT delivers approaches treatment through occupation, and the occupations of a child are different from those of an adult; and include play, chores, selfcare and schoolwork. Common conditions that are specific to or more common in the pediatric population creating a need for OT services include: developmental disorders, sensory regulation or sensory processing deficits, fine motor developmental delays or deficits, autism, emotional and behavioural disturbances (Lambert, 2005), among others. In addition, children are seen for every injury, illness or chronic condition that may cause a person of any age to have performance deficits in their daily life and thus benefit from OT services.

Acute care hospitals: Acute care is an inpatient hospital setting for individuals with a serious medical condition(s) usually due to a traumatic event, such as a traumatic brain injury, spinal cord injury, etc. The primary goal of acute care is to stabilize the patient's medical status and address any threats to his or her life and loss of function. Occupational therapy plays an important role in facilitating early mobilization, restoring function, preventing further decline, and coordinating care, including transition and discharge planning. Furthermore, occupational therapy's role focuses on addressing deficits and barriers that limit the patient's ability to perform activities that they need or want to do related to independence in selfcare, home management, work-related tasks, and participating in leisure and community pursuits.

Inpatient rehabilitation (e.g., Spinal Cord Injuries): People with disabilities have the right and the privilege to live meaningful purposeful lives. When a disability occurs it is sometimes possible to recover – when it is not it is important to learn the skills to adapt capacity and environmental supports to be able to participate. OTs use their knowledge to help both with recovery and adaptation.

Rehabilitation centres (e.g., Traumatic Brain Injury (TBI), Stroke (CVA), Spinal Cord Injuries, Head Injuries)

Skilled nursing facilities: An occupational therapists role in a skilled nursing facility is centered on each client's individual needs. Many of the skills an OT works on are known as activities of daily living or selfcare such as feeding or dressing.

OTs can provide equipment to assist with activities or offer expertise in modifying the environment to maximize independence and facilitate independence. Other OT roles include education in adaptive equipment (shower bench), energy conservation, or task simplification (Hofmann, 2008).

Home Health: Occupational therapists who work in this area of practice generally work with client's in the geriatric population who have one or more of the following diagnoses: Alzheimer's disease, arthritis, depression, CVA, generalized weakness, COPD, or Parkinson's disease. Occupational therapists working with these client's evaluate their level of independence, cognition, and safety. Moreover, occupational therapists provide intervention to maximize independence and function through remedial and compensatory strategies, with the ultimate goal of the client's regaining the ability to live independently at home (Swanson Anderson & Malaski, 1999).

Outpatient clinics (e.g., Hand Therapy, orthopaedics) Hand therapy is a specialty practice area of occupational therapy that is mainly concerned with treating orthopedic-based upper extremity conditions to optimize the functional use of the hand and arm. Diagnoses seen by this practice area include: fractures of the hand or arm, lacerations and amputations, burns, and surgical repairs of tendons and nerves. Additionally, hand therapists treat acquired conditions such as tendonitis, rheumatoid arthritis and osteoarthritis, and carpal tunnel syndrome. Occupational therapists who work in this field address biomechanical issues underlying upper-extremity conditions. In addition, occupational therapists use an occupation-based and client-centered approach by identifying participation needs of the client, then tailoring intervention to improve performance in desired activities.

Hospices: An occupational therapists common role in hospice care is modifying and preventing. Modifying the demands of the activity to fit with the abilities of the client. The intervention may be directly with the client or with the client and the client's caregivers. OT can offer the caregivers support an education. Progress is defined as improved quality of life in hospice care. (Hasselkaus, 1998)

Assisted Living Facilities: In an assisted living facility OT services are provided by a home health agency, rehab agency, or a private practice. Medicare and some private insurance plans cover OT services in ALFs. Areas of treatment intervention often include: bathing, dressing, grooming, toileting, mobility, money management, laundry, and community participation. Can treat persons with occupational performance decline or at risk for a decline. Increase quality of life so less residents need the services of a long-term SNF. Special areas include mobility device assessment (scooter), continence training, psychosocial needs and low vision programs (Fagan, 2001).

Productive Aging: An OT practicing in this area would provide skills and services to older adults to maximize independence, participation, and quality of life. Typical issues addressed: Any impairment or condition that would limit their ability to carry out meaningful occupations and tasks that are necessary for daily life. Skills taught include: energy conservation, education in adaptive equipment (such as a shower bench), task simplification, adapting and modifying activities to progress with a client's changing abilities (Opp Hoffman, 2008), caregiver education and support (AOTA, 2004), safety, social interactions and communication, memory skills training, mobility device assessment and training (i.e. scooters, wheelchairs, walkers), low vision interventions, continence training, and facilitating performance in basic ADL and IADL (Fagan, 2001).

Work hardening is essentially a specialized program designed to enable people with physical, psychological, and psychosocial issues inhibiting a person's ability, to successfully return to work. The National Advisory Committee on Work Hardening best describes work hardening:

"Work hardening is a highly structured, goal oriented, individualized treatment program designed to maximize the individual's ability to return to work. Work hardening programs, which are interdisciplinary in nature, use real or simulated work activities in conjunction with conditioning tasks that are graded to progressively improve the biomechanical, neuromuscular, cardiovascular/metabolic and psychosocial functions of the individual.

Work hardening provides a transition between acute care and return to work while addressing the issues of productivity, safety, physical tolerances, and worker behaviours".

Work conditioning is similar to work hardening, except work conditioning purely involves improving physical capacities, whereas work hardening improves physical, psychological, and psychosocial factors.

Mental Health

According to Medicare (2005) guidance, "Only a qualified occupational therapist has the knowledge, training, and experience required to evaluate and, as necessary, re-evaluate a patient's level of function, determine whether an occupational therapy program could reasonably be expected to improve, restore, or compensate for lost function, and where appropriate, recommend to the physician a plan of treatment."

According to the American Occupational Therapy Association (AOTA), occupational therapists work with the Mental Health population throughout the life span and across many treatment settings where mental health services and psychiatric rehabilitation are provided (AOTA, 2009). Just as with other clients, the OT facilitates maximum independence in activities of daily living (dressing, grooming, etc.) and instrumentaı activities of daily living (medication management, grocery shopping, etc.). According to the American Occupational Therapy Association, OT improves functional capacity and quality of life for people with mental illness in the areas of employment, education, community living, and home and personal care through the use of real life activities in therapy treatments (AOTA, 2005).

Geriatric, Adult, Adolescents, and Children with any kind of mental illness or mental health issues. These conditions include but are not limited to: Schizophrenia, substance abuse, addiction, dementia, Alzheimer's, mood disorders, personality disorders, psychoses, eating disorders, anxiety disorders (including post-traumatic stress disorder, separation anxiety disorder) (Cara & MacRae, 2005), and reactive attachment disorder (children only) (Lambert, 2005).

Typical issues that are addressed are as follows: Helping people acquire the skills to care for themselves or others including; keeping a schedule, medication management, employment, education, increasing community participation, community access (grocery store, library, bank, etc.), money management skills, engaging in productive activities to fill the day, coping skills, routine building, building social skills, and childcare (Cara & MacRae, 2005).

In the UK, the College of Occupational Therapists (COT) have published Recovering Ordinary Lives, which details the strategy for OTs in mental health up to 2017, and makes explicit the goals that have been set for the profession, in line with government directives (COT 2006).

Areas that Mental Health OT's could work in are as follows:

- Mental health inpatient units :
  - o Adolescent, adult and older people's acute mental health wards
  - o Adult and older people's rehabilitation wards
  - o Prisons/secure units (Forensic psychiatry)
  - o Psychiatric intensive care unit
  - o Specialist units for Eating Disorders, Learning disabilities.
- Community based mental health teams :
  - o Child and adolescent mental health teams
  - o Adult and older people's community mental health teams
  - o Rehabilitation and recovery and Assertive Outreach community teams
  - o Primary care services in GP practices
  - o Home treatment teams
  - o early intervention in psychosis teams
  - o Specialist learning disability, eating disorder community services
  - o Day services
  - o Vocational Services.

Dementia & Alzheimer Care: OTs focus on adapting activities as the client progresses through the illness (Hofmann, 2008) OT also works with caregivers to teach them how to grade activities to the client's ability. Interventions are based on using the client's strengths to increase their quality of life and their relationships with caregivers. Use of social interactions, communication, memory, safety and self maintenance.

Community

Community based practice involves working with people in their own environment rather than in a hospital setting. It often combines the knowledge and skills related to physical and mental health. It can also involve working with atypical populations such as the homeless or at-risk populations. Examples of community-based practice settings:

Health promotion and lifestyle change: Remaining healthy is the goal of all people in a society, including people with chronic disabling or health conditions. Achieving health requires skills to self-manage conditions that might limit their ability to function in daily life. The occupational therapist helps people acquire these skills (Wilcock, 2005).

Private Practice

Aging in place: Occupational therapists implement environmental modifications in senior housing, assisted living, long-term-care facilities, and homes (Yamkovenko, 2008) Environmental modifications can include rearranging furniture, building ramps, widening doorways, grab bars, special toilet seats, and other safety equipment to use performance capabilities to their fullest (Moyers & Christiansen, 2004).

Low Vision: Occupational therapists help clients use their remaining vision to complete their daily routines with compensation, remediation, disability prevention and health promotion. Compensations or that modifications to the environment may include proper lighting, color contrast, reducing clutter and education on adaptive equipment (Golembiewski, 2004).

Intermediate Care Services

Driving Centres: Driving is an instrumental activity of daily living and an occupational therapist may evaluate and treat skills needed to drive such as vision, executive function or memory. If a client needs more skilled assessment and training they would refer them to an OT Driver Rehabilitation Specialist which could do on the road assessment, training in adaptive equipment and make more specific recommendations.

- Day centres
- Schools
- Child development centres
- People's own homes, carrying out therapy and providing equipment and adaptations
- Work and Industry: To be a healthy successful worker there must be a person environment fit between the task, the equipment, and the person's skills. Occupational therapists work to achieve that fit. Populations, conditions, and diagnoses: People of working age and ability who have been born with or developed a condition, injury, or illness that compromises their ability to work. Settings: Return to work programs, large organizations, consultants to large organizations, work hardening programs, work conditioning programs, transitional return to work programs. Typical issues addressed: assessment of ability to work, interventions to enhancing work performance by means of work hardening, work conditioning, and improvement of ergonomics in the workplace, identification of accommodations necessary to return-to-work following illness or injury, prevention of work related injury, illness, or disability.
- Homeless Shelters
- Educational Settings
- Refugee Camps

New Emerging Practice Areas for Therapy

- Children & Youth:
  - o Psychosocial Needs of Children & Youth.
- Health & Wellness:
  - o Health & Wellness Consulting
  - o Design & Accessibility Consulting & Home Modification

  - o Ergonomic Consulting
  - o Private Practice Community Health Services
- Productive Aging:
  - o Driver Rehabilitation & Training
  - o Low Vision Services.
- Rehabilitation, Disability, & Participation:
  - o Technology & Assistive Device Development & Consulting.
- Work & Industry:
  - o Ticket to Work Services
  - o Welfare to Work Services.

Occupational Therapy Approaches

Services typically include:

- Teaching new ways of approaching tasks
- How to break down activities into achievable components e.g. sequencing a complex task like cooking a complex meal
- Comprehensive home and job site evaluations with adaptation recommendations.
- Performance skills assessments and treatment.
- Adaptive equipment recommendations and usage training.
- Environmental adaptation including provision of equipment or designing adaptations to remove obstacles or make them manageable
- Guidance to family members and caregivers.
- The use of creative media as therapeutic activity

Activity Analysis

Activity analysis has been defined as a process of dissecting an activity into its component parts and task sequence in order to identify its inherent properties and the skills required for its performance, thus allowing the therapist to evaluate its therapeutic potential

Theoretical Frameworks

Occupational Therapists use a number of theoretical frameworks to frame their practice. Note that terminology has differed between scholars. Theoretical bases for framing a human and their occupation being include the following:

Frames of Reference/Generic Models

Frames of reference or generic models are the overarching title given to a collation of compatible knowledge, research and theories that form conceptual practice. More generally they can be defined as "those aspects which influence our perceptions, decisions and practice".

Occupational Therapy Frame of References/Models:

- Person Environment Occupation Performance Model (PEOP)
- Occupational Performance Model (OPM)
- Model of Human Occupation (MOHO)
- Canadian Model of Occupational Performance (CMOP)
- Biomechanical
- Rehabilitative (compensatory)
- Neurofunctional (Gordon Muir Giles and Clark-Wilson)
- Cognitive Disabilities
- Sensory Integration
- Lifestyle Performance Model (Fidler).

Challenges for Occupational Therapy

A key challenge for occupational therapy is to develop and maintain a definition of its nature and scope assert that while this presents a challenge, it also results in a unique flexibility which allows the discipline to move with the flow of social, cultural and environmental change. This difficulty in definition may be a cause of chronic strain for practitioners and may also contribute to a lack of role definition and subsequent blurring.

Recent literature has also called for occupational therapy to address the political nature of who occupational therapists are and what they do. Profession specific models of occupational therapy have also been critiqued for being biased towards a western, ableist and generally unrepresentative of the most occupationally deprived groups.

Occupational Therapy and ICF

The International Classification of Functioning, Disability and Health (ICF) is an outcome measure for health and occupation and illustrates how these components impact one's function. This relates very closely to the Occupational Therapy Practice Framework as it is stated, "The profession's core beliefs are in the positive relationship between occupation and health and its view of people as occupational beings" (2008). The ICF is also built into the 2nd edition of the practice framework. Activities and participation examples from the ICF overlap Areas of Occupation, Performance Skills, and Performance Patterns in the framework. The ICF also includes contextual factors (environmental and personal factors) that relate to the context in the framework. In addition, Body functions and structures classified within the ICF help describe the client factors as described in the OT framework (AOTA, 2002).

Further exploration of the relationship between occupational therapy and the components of the ICIDH-2 (revision of the original International Classification of Impairments, Disabilities, and Handicaps (ICIDH); later becoming the ICF) was conducted by McLaughlin Gray (2001). First, the ICF is an international framework and provides an opportunity for the occupational therapy field to become better known across the globe. Second, the ICF provides occupational therapists with a global language to describe their expertise to the larger international health care community. The ICF uses a positive, holistic language emphasizing skills, capacities, and strengths of an individual rather than focusing on one's deficits and disabilities. This is similar to the outlook of occupational therapists. Third, the ICF includes environmental and personal contextual factors which are incorporated into the theory behind occupational therapy. It is important to take into consideration an individual's personal, environmental, and occupational factors to develop an effective intervention (Christiansen & Baum, 2005). The last notable application of the

ICF to occupational therapy is the recognition of cultural patterns in occupation. Culture has significance on an individual's activities and participation and it is important to keep this in mind when treating an individual.

Although the ICF can be very useful for occupational therapists, it is noted in the literature that occupational therapists should use specific occupational therapy vocabulary along with the ICF in order to ensure correct communication about specific concepts. The ICF might lack certain categories to describe what occupational therapists need to communicate to clients and colleagues. It also may not be possible to exactly match the connotations of the ICF categories to occupational therapy terms. The ICF is not an assessment and specialized occupational therapy vocabulary should not be replaced with ICF terminology. (Haglund & Henriksson, 2003). The ICF is an overarching framework on which to hang current therapy practices.

Trauma Centre

A trauma centre is a hospital equipped to provide comprehensive emergency medical services to patients suffering traumatic injuries. Trauma centres were established as the medical establishment realized that traumatic injuries often require complex and multi-disciplinary treatment, including surgery in order to give the victim the best possible chance for survival and recovery.

According to the CDC, injuries are the leading cause of death for children and adults ages 1–44.

Trauma is any life-threatening occurrence, either accidental or intentional, that causes injuries. The leading causes of trauma are motor vehicle accidents, falls, and assaults. Moreover, trauma (or injury) is the leading cause of death among Americans under 44 years of age.

In order to qualify as a trauma centre in America, a hospital must meet certain criteria as established by the American College of Surgeons (ACS). Trauma centres vary in their specific capabilities and are identified by "Level" designation: Level-I (Level-1) being the highest, to Level-III (Level-3) being the lowest (some states have four designated levels, in which case Level-IV (Level-4) is the lowest). Higher levels of trauma centres will have trauma surgeons available, including those trained in such specialties as Neurosurgery and Orthopedic surgery as well as highly sophisticated medical diagnostic equipment. Lower levels of trauma centres may only be able to provide initial care and stabilization of a traumatic injury and arrange for transfer of the victim to a higher level of trauma care.

The operation of a trauma centre is extremely expensive. Some areas are under-served by trauma centres because of this expense (for example, Harborview Medical Centre in Seattle is the only Level I trauma centre to serve the entirety of Washington, Idaho, Montana, and Alaska). As there is no way to schedule the need for emergency services, patient traffic at trauma centres can vary widely. A variety of different methods have been developed for dealing with this. Halifax Health in Daytona Beach, Florida will soon deploy a "pod system," allowing trauma care to be provided by several different small Emergency Departments at different hospitals, rather than at one central large trauma centre.

A trauma centre will often have a helipad for receiving patients that have been airlifted to the hospital. In many cases, persons injured in remote areas and transported to a distant trauma centre by helicopter can receive faster and better medical care than if they had been transported by ground ambulance to a closer hospital which is not a designated trauma centre.

History

The concept of a trauma centre was developed at the University of Maryland, Baltimore in the 1960s and 1970s by heart surgeon and shock researcher R Adams Cowley, who founded what became the Shock Trauma Centre in Baltimore, Maryland in 1961. Cook County Hospital in Chicago, Illinois claims to be the first trauma centre (opened in 1966) in the United States. Dr. David R Boyd interned at Cook County Hospital from 1963-1964 before being drafted into the United States Army. Upon his release from the Army, Dr. Boyd became the first shock-trauma fellow at the Shock Trauma Centre from 1967-1968. Dr. Boyd returned to Cook County Hospital, where he went on to serve as resident director of the Cook County Trauma Unit.

Definitions in the United States

In the United States, trauma centres are ranked by the American College of Surgeons (ACS), from Level I (comprehensive service) to Level III (limited-care). The different levels refer to the kinds of resources available in a trauma centre and the number of patients admitted yearly. These are categories that define national standards for trauma care in hospitals. Level I and Level II designations are also given adult and or pediatric designations. Additionally, some states have their own trauma centre rankings separate from the ACS. These levels may range from Level I to Level IV.

Level I

A Level I trauma centre provides the highest level of surgical care to trauma patients. It has a full range of specialists and equipment available 24 hours a day and admits a minimum required annual volume of severely injured patients. A Level I trauma centre is required to have a certain number of surgeons and anesthesiologists on duty 24 hours a day at the hospital, an education program, preventive and outreach programs. Key elements include 24-hour in-house coverage by general surgeons and prompt availability of care in varying specialties such as orthopedic surgery, neurosurgery, plastic surgery (plastic surgeons often take calls for hand and facial injuries fixing both the bone and soft tissue of these specialized regions), anesthesiology, emergency medicine, radiology, internal medicine, oral and maxillofacial surgery, and critical care, which are needed to adequately respond and care for various forms of trauma that a patient may suffer. Additionally, a Level I centre has a program of research, is a leader in trauma education and injury prevention, and is a referral resource for communities in nearby regions.

Level I trauma centre hospitals in most states in the U.S. (New York, and Pennsylvania among others are notable exceptions) are designated by the American College of Surgeons (ACS) for a period of three years. Pennsylvania has its own rankings system, based on the criteria of the Commonwealth's Trauma Foundation.

The ACS does not *officially* designate hospitals as regional trauma centres, however. Numerous U.S. hospitals that are not listed on the organization's trauma roster nevertheless refer to their emergency or trauma units as "Level I trauma centres." The ACS describes that responsibility as "a geopolitical process by which empowered entities, government or otherwise, are authorized to designate." The ACS's self-appointed mission is limited to confirming and reporting on any given hospital's ability to comply with the ACS standard of care known as *Resources for Optimal Care of the Injured Patient.*

Level II

A Level II trauma centre works in collaboration with a Level I centre. It provides comprehensive trauma care and supplements the clinical expertise of a Level I institution. It provides 24-hour availability of all essential specialties, personnel, and equipment. Minimum volume requirements may depend on local conditions. These institutions are not required to have an ongoing program of research or a surgical residency program.

Level III

A Level III trauma centre does not have the full availability of specialists, but does have resources for emergency resuscitation, surgery, and intensive care of most trauma patients. A Level III centre has transfer agreements with Level I or Level II trauma centres that provide back-up resources for the care of exceptionally severe injuries, Example: Rural or Community hospitals.

Level IV

A Level IV trauma centre exists in some states where the resources do not exist for a Level III trauma centre. It provides initial evaluation, stabilization, diagnostic capabilities, and transfer to a higher level of care. It may also provide surgery and critical care services as defined in the scope of services of trauma care. A trauma trained nurse is immediately available, and physicians are available upon the patients arrival to the Emergency Department. Transfer agreements exist with other trauma centres with higher levels when conditions warrant a transfer.

Post Anesthesia Care Unit

A post anesthesia care unit, often abbreviated PACU and sometimes referred to as post anesthesia recovery or PAR, is a vital part of hospitals, ambulatory care centres, and other medical facilities. It is an area, normally attached to operating theatre suites, designed to provide care for patients recovering from anesthesia, whether it be general anaesthesia, regional anaesthesia, or local anesthesia.

Common Activities

The PACU staff, generally composed of highly trained nurses are charged with many vital tasks for the care of post-anaesthesia and post-operative patients. These essential activities include:-

- monitoring vital signs (heart rate, blood pressure, temperature and respiratory rate)
- managing post-operative pain.
- treating symptoms of postoperative nausea and vomiting (or PONV)
- monitoring surgical site(s) for excessive bleeding, discharge, swelling, hematoma, redness, etc.

These common activities may often need supplementing with more intensive care or treatment. This may require :

- Preparation and education for the use of Patient Controlled Analgesia (PCA) units
- Preparation and establishment of IV, epidural or perineural infusions
- Preparation and establishment of invasive monitoring such as arterial lines, central venous lines, ventriculostomies, etc.

Post-Operative Complications

Occasionally, serious life threatening complications, such as laryngospasm or respiratory arrest, can arise post-anesthesia. Patients are cared for with interdisciplinary measures from Anesthesiologists, Certified Nurse Anesthetists or CRNA's, PACU nurses and Surgeons. Patients may remain or have to be re-intubated due to anaphylaxis, pulmonary edema, pneumothorax, or complications from surgery such as extended operative time and long-term exposure to anesthesia and narcotics. Unless complications occur, most patients will only stay in the PACU for a few hours, before returning home or to another department of the hospital.

Certification

PACU nurses can be certified in their field by obtaining ASPAN (American Society of Perianesthesia Nurses) certification, either by getting their CPAN or Certified PostAnesthesia Nurse or CAPA (Certified Ambulatory Perianesthesia Nurse) certification(s). Both can be achieved by one person.

Psychiatric Hospital

Psychiatric hospitals, also known as mental hospitals, are hospitals specializing in the treatment of serious mental disorder.

Psychiatric hospitals vary widely in their goals and methods. Some hospitals may specialize only in short-term or outpatient therapy for low-risk patients. Others may specialize in the temporary or permanent care of residents who as a result of a psychological disorder, require routine assistance, treatment or a specialized and controlled environment. Patients are often admitted on a voluntary basis, but involuntary commitment is practiced when an individual may pose a significant danger to themselves or others.

History

Modern psychiatric hospitals evolved from, and eventually replaced the older lunatic asylums. The development of the modern psychiatric hospital is also the story of the rise of organised, institutional psychiatry. While there were earlier institutions that housed the 'insane' the arrival at the answer of institutionalisation as the correct solution to the problem of madness was very much an event of the nineteenth century. To illustrate this with one regional example, in England at the beginning of the nineteenth century there were, perhaps, a few thousand 'lunatics' housed in a variety of disparate institutions but by 1900 that figure had grown to about 100,000. That this growth coincided with the growth of alienism, later known as psychiatry, as a medical specialism is not coincidental.

The treatment of inmates in lunatic asylums was often brutal, focused on containment and restraint. With successive waves of reform, and the introduction of effective evidence-based treatments, modern psychiatric hospitals provide a primary emphasis on treatment, and attempt where possible to help patients control their own lives in the outside world, with the aid of a combination of psychiatric drugs and psychotherapy.

Types

There are a number of different types of modern psychiatric hospitals, but all of them house people with mental illnesses of widely variable severity.

Crisis Stabilization

The crisis stabilization unit is in effect an emergency room for psychiatry, frequently dealing with suicidal, violent, or otherwise critical individuals. Laws in many jurisdictions providing for long term involuntary commitment require a commitment order issued by a judge within a short time (after 72 hours, the evaluation period) of the patient's entry to the unit, if the patient does not or is unable to consent themselves.

Open Units

Open units are psychiatric units that are less secure than crisis stabilization units. They are not used for acutely suicidal persons; the focus in these units is to make life as normal as possible for patients while continuing treatment to the point where they can be discharged. However, patients are usually still not allowed to hold their own medications in their rooms, because of the risk of an impulsive overdose. While some open units are physically unlocked, other open units still use locked entrances and exits depending on the type of patients admitted.

Medium-term

Another type of psychiatric hospital is a medium term, which provides care lasting several weeks. Most drugs used for psychiatric purposes take several weeks to take effect, and the main purpose of these hospitals is to monitor the patient for the first few weeks of therapy to ensure the treatment is effective.

Juvenile Wards

Juvenile wards are sections of psychiatric hospitals or psychiatric wards set aside for children and/or adolescents with mental illness. However, there are a number of institutions specializing only in the treatment of juveniles, particularly when dealing with drug abuse, self harm, or eating disorders.

Long Term Care Facilities

In the UK long-term care facilities are now being replaced with smaller secure units (some within the hospitals listed above). Modern buildings, modern security and being locally sited to help with reintegration into society once medication has stabilized the condition are often features of such units. An example of this is the Three Bridges Unit, in the grounds of Hanwell Asylum in West London and the John Munroe Hospital in Staffordshire. However these modern units have the goal of treatment and rehabilitation back into society within a short time-frame (two or three years) and not all forensic patients' treatment can meet this criterion, so the large hospitals mentioned above often retain this role. These hospitals provide stabalization and rehabilitation for those who are having difficulties such as depression, eating disorders, mental disorders, and so on.

Halfway Houses

One type of institution for the mentally ill is a community-based halfway house. These facilities provide assisted living for patients with mental illnesses for an extended period of time, and often aid in the transition to self-sufficiency. These institutions are considered to be one of the most important parts of a mental health system by many psychiatrists, although some localities lack sufficient funding.

Political Imprisonment

In some countries the mental institution may be used for the incarceration of political prisoners, as a form of punishment.

Anti-psychiatry Objections

Some critics, notably psychiatrist Dr. Thomas Szasz, have objected to calling mental hospitals "hospitals".

The French historian Michel Foucault is widely known for his comprehensive critique of the use and abuse of the mental hospital system in *Madness and Civilization*. He argued that Tuke and Pinel's asylum was a symbolic recreation of the condition of a child under a bourgeois family. It was a microcosm symbolizing the massive structures of bourgeois society and its values: relations of Family-Children (paternal authority), Fault-Punishment (immediate justice), Madness-Disorder (social and moral order).

Erving Goffman coined the term 'Total Institution' for places which took over and confined a person's whole life. The anti-psychiatry movement coming to the fore in the 1960s oppose many of the practices, conditions, or existence of mental hospitals. The Consumer/Survivor Movement has often objected to or campaigned against conditions in mental hospitals or their use, voluntarily or involuntarily.

Some anti-psychiatry activists have advocated for the abolition of long-term hospitals for the criminally insane, including on the grounds that those judged not guilty by reason of insanity should not then be indefinitely confined with potentially less legal rights, or on the converse grounds that insanity is not a coherent concept and so should not be a basis for different treatment.

Medical Record

A medical record, health record, or medical chart is a systematic documentation of a patient's medical history and care. The term 'Medical record' is used both for the physical folder for each individual patient and for the body of information which comprises the total of each patient's health history. Medical records are intensely personal documents and there are many ethical and legal issues surrounding them such as the degree of third-party access and appropriate storage and disposal. Although medical records are traditionally compiled and stored by health care providers, personal health records maintained by individual patients have become more popular in recent years.

Purpose

The information contained in the medical record allows health care providers to provide continuity of care to individual patients.

The medical record also serves as a basis for planning patient care, documenting communication between the health care provider and any other health professional contributing to the patient's care, assisting in protecting the legal interest of the patient and the health care providers responsible for the patient's care, and documenting the care and services provided to the patient. In addition, the medical record may serve as a document to educate medical students/resident physicians, to provide data for internal hospital auditing and quality assurance, and to provide data for medical research. Personal health records combine many of the above features with portability, thus allowing a patient to share medical records across providers and health care systems.

Format

Traditionally, medical records have been written on paper and kept in folders. These folders are typically divided into useful sections, with new information added to each section chronologically as the patient experiences new medical issues. Active records are usually housed at the clinical site, but older records (e.g., those of the deceased) are often kept in separate facilities.

The advent of electronic medical records has not only changed the format of medical records but has increased accessibility of files. The use of an individual dossier style medical record, where records are kept on each patient by name and illness type originated at the Mayo Clinic out of a desire to simplify patient tracking and to allow for medical research.

Contents

Although the specific content of the medical record may vary depending upon specialty and location, it usually contains the patient's identification information, the patient's health history (what the patient tells the healthcare providers about his or her past and present health status), and the patient's medical examination findings (what the healthcare providers observe when the patient is examined). Other information may include lab test results; medications prescribed; referrals ordered to healthcare providers; educational materials provided; and what plans there are for further care, including patient instruction for selfcare and return visits. In some places, billing information is considered to be part of the medical record.

Demographics

Demographics include patient information that is not medical in nature. It is often information to locate the patient, including identifying numbers, addresses, and contact numbers. It may contain information about race and religion as well as workplace and type of occupation. It may also contain information regarding the patient's health insurance.

Medical History

The medical history is a longitudinal record of what has happened to the patient since birth. It chronicles diseases, major and minor illnesses, as well as growth landmarks. It gives the clinician a feel for what has happened before to the patient. As a result, it may often give clues to current disease states.

Surgical History

The surgical history is a chronicle of surgery performed for the patient. It may have dates of operations, operative reports, and/or the detailed narrative of what the surgeon did.

Obstetric History

The obstetric history lists prior pregnancies and their outcomes. It also includes any complications of these pregnancies.

Medications and medical allergies

The medical record may contain a summary of the patient's current and previous medications as well as any medical allergies.

Family History

The family history lists the health status of immediate family members as well as their causes of death (if known). It may also list diseases common in the family or found only in one sex or the other. It may also include a pedigree chart. It is a valuable asset in predicting some outcomes for the patient.

Social History

The social history is a chronicle of human interactions. It tells of the relationships of the patient, his/her careers and trainings, schooling and religious training. It is helpful for the physician to know what sorts of community support the patient might expect during a major illness. It may explain the behavior of the patient in relation to illness or loss. It may also give clues as to the cause of an illness (e.g. occupational exposure to asbestos).

Habits

Various habits which impact health, such as tobacco use, alcohol intake, exercise, and diet are chronicled, often as part of the social history. This section may also include more intimate details such as sexual habits and sexual orientation.

Medical Encounters

Within the medical record, individual medical encounters are marked by discrete summations of a patient's medical history by a physician, nurse practitioner, or physician assistant and can take several forms. Hospital admission documentation (i.e., when a patient requires hospitalization) or consultation by a specialist often take an exhaustive form, detailing the entirety of prior health and health care. Routine visits by a provider familiar to the patient, however, may take a shorter form such as the *problem-oriented medical record* (POMR), which includes a problem list of diagnoses or a "SOAP" method of documentation for each visit. Each encounter will generally contain the aspects below:

Chief Complaint

This is the problem that has brought the patient to see the doctor. Information on the nature and duration of the problem will be explored.

History of the present illness: A detailed exploration of the symptoms the patient is experiencing that have caused the patient to seek medical attention.

Physical examination: The physical examination is the recording of observations of the patient. This includes the vital signs , muscle power and examination of the different organ systems, especially ones that might directly be responsible for the symptoms the patient is experiencing.

Assessment and plan: The assessment is a written summation of what are the most likely causes of the patient's current set of symptoms. The plan documents the expected course of action to address the symptoms (diagnosis, treatment, etc.).

Orders

Written orders by medical providers are included in the medical record. These detail the instructions given to other members of the health care team by the primary providers.

Progress notes

When a patient is hospitalized, daily updates are entered into the medical record documenting clinical changes, new information, etc. These often take the form of a SOAP note and are entered by all members of the healthcare team (doctors, nurses, physical therapists, dietitians, clinical pharmacists, respiratory therapists, etc.). They are kept in chronological order and document the sequence of events leading to the current state of health.

Test Results

The results of testing, such as blood tests (e.g., complete blood count) radiology examinations (e.g., X-rays), pathology (e.g., biopsy results), or specialized testing (e.g., pulmonary function testing) are included. Often, as in the case of X-rays, a written report of the findings is included in lieu of the actual film.

Other Information

Many other items are variably kept within the medical record. Digital images of the patient, flowsheets from operations/intensive care units, informed consent forms, EKG tracings, outputs from medical devices (such as pacemakers), chemotherapy protocols, and numerous other important pieces of information form part of the record depending on the patient and his or her set of illnesses/ treatments.

There are several information needed to be recorded while tracing state of patient's daily health:

1. Vital Signs: Body Temperature, Pulse Rate(Heart Rate), Blood Pressure and Respiratory Rate.
2. Intake: Medication, Fluid, Nutrition, Water and Blood, etc.
3. Output: Blood, Urine, Excrement, Vomitus and Sweat, etc.
4. Observation on Pupil size.
5. Capability of four limbs of body.

Administrative Issues

Medical records are legal documents and are subject to the laws of the country/state in which they are produced. As such, there is great variability in rule governing production, ownership, accessibility, and destruction.

Production

In the United States, written records must be marked with the date and time and scribed with indelible pens without use of corrective paper. Errors in the record should be struck out with a single line and initialed by the author. Orders and notes must be signed by the author. Electronic versions require an electronic signature.

Ownership

In the United States, the data contained within the medical record belongs to the patient, whereas the physical form the data takes belongs to the entity responsible for maintaining the record (Health Insurance Portability and Accountability Act). Therefore, patients have the right to ensure that the information contained in their record is accurate. Patients can petition their health care provider to remedy factually incorrect information in their records.

In the United Kingdom, ownership of the NHS's medical records belong to the Department of Health, and this is taken by some to mean copyright also belongs to the authorities.

Accessibility

In the United States, the most basic rules governing access to a medical record dictate that only the patient and the healthcare providers directly involved in delivering care have the right to view the record. The patient, however, may grant consent for any person or entity to evaluate the record. The full rules regarding access and security for medical records are set forth under the guidelines of the Health Insurance Portability and Accountability Act (HIPAA). The rules become more complicated in special situations.

Capacity

When a patient does not have capacity (is not legally able) to make decisions regarding his or her own care, a legal guardian is designated (either through next of kin or by action of a court of law if no kin exists). Legal guardians have the ability to access the medical record in order to make medical decisions on the patient's behalf. Those without capacity include the comatose, minors (unless emancipated), and patients with incapacitating psychiatric illness or intoxication.

Medical Emergency

In the event of a medical emergency involving a non-communicative patient, consent to access medical records is assumed unless written documentation has been previously drafted (such as an advance directive)

Research, Auditing, and Evaluation

Individuals involved in medical research, financial or management audits, or program evaluation have access to the medical record. They are not allowed access to any identifying information, however.

Risk of Death or Harm

Information within the record can be shared with authorities without permission when failure to do so would result in death or harm, either to the patient or to others. Information cannot be used, however, to initiate or substantiate a charge unless the previous criteria are met (i.e., information from illicit drug testing cannot be used to bring charges of possession against a patient). This rule was established in the United States Supreme Court case Jaffe v. Redmond.

In the United Kingdom, the Data Protection Acts and later the Freedom of Information Act 2000 gave patients or their representatives the right to a copy of their record, except where information breaches confidentiality (e.g., information from another family member or where a patient has asked for information not to be disclosed to third parties) or would be harmful to the patient's wellbeing (e.g., some psychiatric assessments). Also, the legislation gives patients the right to check for any errors in their record and insist that amendments be made if required.

Destruction

In general, entities in possession of medical records are required to maintain those records for a given period. In the United Kingdom, medical records are required for the lifetime of a patient and legally for as long as that complaint action can be brought. Generally in the UK, any recorded information should be kept legally for 7 years, but for medical records additional time must be allowed for any child to reach the age of responsibility (20 years). Medical records are required many years after a patient's death to investigate illnesses within a community (e.g., industrial or environmental disease or even deaths at the hands of doctors committing murders, as in the Harold Shipman case).

Abuses

- The outsourcing of medical record transcription and storage has the potential to violate patient-physician confidentiality by possibly allowing unaccountable persons access to patient data.
- Falsification of a medical record by a medical professional is a felony in most United States jurisdictions.
- Governments have often refused to disclose medical records of military personnel who have been used as experimental subjects.

Release of Information Department

A release of information (ROI) department or division is found in virtually every hospital. In the United States, HIPAA and State guidelines strongly direct the rules and regulations of patient information. ROI departments perform such tasks as obtaining patient consent, certifying medical records, and deciding what information can be released.

The ROI department is often found within the health information management services (HIMS) department of a hospital. The oversight of the HIMS department is usually overseen by a director. The director of health information may have credentials such as RHIT (registered health information technician) or RHIA (registered health information administrator).

Special federal regulations protect the release of information in the areas of mental health, drug treatment, and alcohol treatment. Records of this nature often require either a patient's consent or a court order for their release. ROI staff must possess a strong acumen for the legal rights of the patient.

History

Early Examples

In ancient cultures, religion and medicine were linked. The earliest documented institutions aiming to provide cures were Egyptian temples. In ancient Greece, temples dedicated to the healer-god Asclepius, known as *Asclepieia* , functioned as centres of medical advice, prognosis, and healing. At these shrines, patients would enter a dream-like state of induced sleep known as "enkoimesis" not unlike anesthesia, in which they either received guidance from the deity in a dream or were cured by surgery. Asclepeia provided carefully controlled spaces conducive to healing and fulfilled several of the requirements of institutions created for healing. In the Asclepieion of Epidaurus, three large marble boards dated to 350 BC preserve the names, case histories, complaints, and cures of about 70 patients who came to the temple with a problem and shed it there.

Some of the surgical cures listed, such as the opening of an abdominal abscess or the removal of traumatic foreign material, are realistic enough to have taken place, but with the patient in a state of enkoimesis induced with the help of soporific substances such as opium. The worship of Asclepius was adopted by the Romans. Under his Roman name Æsculapius, he was provided with a temple (291 BC) on an island in the Tiber in Rome, where similar rites were performed.

According to the Mahavamsa, the ancient chronicle of Sinhalese royalty, written in the sixth century A.D., King Pandukabhaya (fourth century B.C.) had lying-in-homes and hospitals (Sivikasotthi-Sala) built in various parts of the country. This is the earliest documentary evidence we have of institutions specifically dedicated to the care of the sick anywhere in the world. Mihintale Hospital is the oldest in the world. Ruins of ancient hospitals in Sri Lanka are still in existence in Mihintale, Anuradhapura, and Medirigiriya.

Institutions created specifically to care for the ill also appeared early in India. King Ashoka is said to have founded at least eighteen hospitals ca. 230 B.C., with physicians and nursing staff, the expense being borne by the royal treasury. Stanley Finger (2001) in his book, *Origins of Neuroscience: A History of Explorations Into Brain Function*, cites an Ashokan edict translated as: "Everywhere King Piyadasi (Asoka) erected two kinds of hospitals, hospitals for people and hospitals for animals. Where there were no healing herbs for people and animals, he ordered that they be bought and planted." However Dominik Wujastyk of the University College London disputes this, arguing that the edict indicates that Ashoka built rest houses (for travellers) instead of hospitals, and that this was misinterpreted due to the reference to medical herbs.

The first teaching hospital where students were authorized to practice methodically on patients under the supervision of physicians as part of their education, was the Academy of Gundishapur in the Persian Empire. One expert has argued that "to a very large extent, the credit for the whole hospital system must be given to Persia".

Roman Empire

The Romans created *valetudinaria* for the care of sick slaves, gladiators, and soldiers around 100 B.C., and many were identified by later archeology. While their existence is considered proven, there is some doubt as to whether they were as widespread as was once thought, as many were identified only according to the layout of building remains, and not by means of surviving records or finds of medical tools.

The adoption of Christianity as the state religion of the Roman Empire drove an expansion of the provision of care. The First Council of Nicaea in 325 A.D. urged the church to provide for the poor, sick, widows, and strangers. It ordered the construction of a hospital in every cathedral town. Among the earliest were those built by the physician Saint Sampson in Constantinople and by Basil, bishop of Caesarea. The latter was attached to a monastery and provided lodgings for poor and travelers, as well as treating the sick and infirm. There was a separate section for lepers.

Medieval Islamic World

In the medieval Islamic world, the word "bimaristan" was used to indicate a hospital establishment where the ill were welcomed, cared for and treated by qualified staff. In this way medieval Islamic physicians distinguished between a hospital and earlier ancient establishments such as a healing temple, sleep temple, hospice, asylum, lazaret, or leper-house, all of which were common in antiquity and more concerned with isolating the sick and the mad (insane) from society than offering them a true cure. Some thus consider the medieval Bimaristan hospitals as "the first hospitals" in the modern sense of the word.

The first free public hospital in Baghdad was opened during the Abbasid Caliphate of Harun al-Rashid in the 8th century. The first hospital in Egypt was opened in 872 and thereafter public hospitals sprang up all over the empire from Islamic Spain and the Maghrib to Persia. As the system developed, physicians and surgeons were appointed who gave lectures to medical students and issued diplomas to those who were considered qualified to practice, an early parallel to modern medical schools. The first psychiatric hospital was built in Baghdad in 705. Many other Islamic hospitals also often had their own wards dedicated to mental health.

Between the eighth and twelfth centuries CE Muslim hospitals developed a high standard of care. Hospitals in Baghdad in the ninth and tenth centuries employed up to twenty-five staff physicians and had separate wards for different conditions. Al-Qairawan hospital and mosque, in Tunisia, were built under the Aghlabid rule in 830 CE and was simple, but adequately equipped with halls organized into waiting rooms, a mosque, and a special bath. The hospital employed female nurses, including nurses from Sudan. In addition to regular physicians who attended the sick, there were *Fuqaha al-Badan*, a kind of religious physio-therapists, group of religious scholars whose medical services included bloodletting, bone setting, and cauterisation. During Ottoman rule, when hospitals reached a particular distinction, Sultan Bayazid II built a psychiatric hospital and medical madrasa in Edirne, and a number of other early hospitals also were built in Turkey.

Medieval Europe

Medieval hospitals in Europe followed a similar pattern to the Byzantine. They were religious communities, with care provided by monks and nuns. (An old French term for hospital is *hotel-Dieu*, "hostel of God.") Some were attached to monasteries; others were independent and had their own endowments, usually of property, which provided income for their support. Some hospitals were multi-functional while others were founded for specific purposes such as leper hospitals, or as refuges for the poor, or for pilgrims: not all cared for the sick. The first Spanish hospital, founded by the Catholic Visigoth bishop Masona in 580 at Merida, was a *xenodochium* designed as an inn for travellers (mostly pilgrims to the shrine of Eulalia of Mérida) as well as a hospital for citizens and local farmers. The hospital's endowment consisted of farms to feed its patients and guests.

Colonial America

The first hospital founded in the Americas was the Hospital San Nicolas de Bari [Calle Hostos] in Santo Domingo, Distrito Nacional Dominican Republic. Fray Nicolas de Ovando, Spanish governor and colonial administrator from 1502–1509, authorized its construction on December 29, 1503. This hospital apparently incorporated a church. The first phase of its construction was completed in 1519, and it was rebuilt in 1552. Abandoned in the mid-eighteenth century, the hospital now lies in ruins near the Cathedral in Santo Domingo.

Conquistador Hernan Cortes founded the two earliest hospitals in North America: the Immaculate Conception Hospital and the Saint Lazarus Hospital. The oldest was the Immaculate Conception, now the Hospital de Jesus Nazareno in Mexico City, founded in 1524 to care for the poor.

The first hospital north of Mexico was the Hotel-Dieu de Quebec. It was established in New France in 1639 by three Augustinians from Hotel-Dieu de Dieppe in France. The project, begun by the niece of Cardinal de Richelieu was granted a royal charter by King Louis XIII and staffed by colonial physician Robert Giffard de Moncel.

Modern Era

In Europe the medieval concept of Christian care evolved during the sixteenth and seventeenth centuries into a secular one, but it was in the eighteenth century that the modern hospital began to appear, serving only medical needs and staffed with physicians and surgeons. The Charite (founded in Berlin in 1710) is an early example.

Guy's Hospital was founded in London in 1724 from a bequest by the wealthy merchant, Thomas Guy. Other hospitals sprang up in London and other British cities over the century, many paid for by private subscriptions. In the British American colonies the Pennsylvania General Hospital was chartered in Philadelphia in 1751, after £2,000 from private subscription was matched by funds from the Assembly.

When the Vienna General Hospital opened in 1784 (instantly becoming the world's largest hospital), physicians acquired a new facility that gradually developed into the most important research centre. During the nineteenth century, the Second Viennese Medical School emerged with the contributions of physicians such as Carl Freiherr von Rokitansky, Josef Skoda, Ferdinand Ritter von Hebra, and Ignaz Philipp Semmelweis. Basic medical science expanded and specialization advanced. Furthermore, the first dermatology, eye, as well as ear, nose, and throat clinics in the world were founded in Vienna, being considered as the birth of specialized medicine.

By the mid-nineteenth century most of Europe and the United States had established a variety of public and private hospital systems. In continental Europe the new hospitals generally were built and run from public funds. The National Health Service, the principle provider of health care in the United Kingdom, was founded in 1948.

In the United States the traditional hospital is a non-profit hospital, usually sponsored by a religious denomination. One of the earliest of these "almshouses" in what would become the United States was started by William Penn in Philadelphia in 1713. These hospitals are tax-exempt due to their charitable purpose, but provide only a minimum of charitable medical care. They are supplemented by large public hospitals in major cities and research hospitals often affiliated with a medical school. The largest public hospital system in America is the New York City Health and Hospitals Corporation, which includes Bellevue Hospital, the oldest U.S. hospital, affiliated with New York University Medical School. In the late twentieth century, chains of for-profit hospitals arose in the USA.

Criticism

While hospitals, by concentrating equipment, skilled staff and other resources in one place, clearly provide important help to patients with serious or rare health problems, hospitals also are criticised for a number of faults, some of which are endemic to the system, others which develop from what some consider wrong approaches to health care.

One criticism often voiced is the 'industrialised' nature of care, with constantly shifting treatment staff, which dehumanises the patient and prevents more effective care as doctors and nurses rarely are intimately familiar with the patient. The high working pressures often put on the staff exacerbate such rushed and impersonal treatment. The architecture and setup of modern hospitals often is voiced as a contributing factor to the feelings of faceless treatment many people complain about.

Another criticism is that hospitals are in themselves dangerous places for patients, who are often suffering from weakened immune systems - either due to their body having to undergo substantial surgery or because of the illness which placed them in the hospital itself. Most of these criticisms stem from the pre-Listerian era. However, even in modern hospitals, hospital-acquired infections can be an important cause of hospital related morbidity, and sometimes mortality.

Funding

In the modern era, hospitals are, broadly, either funded by the government of the country in which they are situated, or survive financially by competing in the private sector (a number of hospitals also are still supported by the historical type of charitable or religious associations).

In the United Kingdom for example, a relatively comprehensive, "free at the point of delivery" health care system exists, funded by the state. Hospital care is thus relatively easily available to all legal residents (although as hospitals prioritize their limited resources, there is a tendency for 'waiting lists' for non-emergency treatment in countries with such systems, and those who can afford it, often take out private health care to get treatment more quickly). On the other hand, many countries, including for example the USA, have in the twentieth century followed a largely private-based, for-profit-approach to providing hospital care, with few state-money supported 'charity' hospitals remaining today. Where for-profit hospitals in such countries admit uninsured patients in emergency situations (such as during and after Hurricane Katrina in the USA), they incur direct financial losses, ensuring that there is a clear disincentive to admit such patients.

As quality of health care has increasingly become an issue around the world, hospitals have increasingly had to pay serious attention to this. Independent external assessment of quality is one of the most powerful ways of assessing the quality of health care, and hospital accreditation is one means by which this is achieved. In many parts of the world such accreditation is sourced from other countries, a phenomenon known as international health care accreditation, by groups such as Accreditation Canada from Canada, the Joint Commission from the USA, the Trent

Accreditation Scheme from Great Britain, and Haute Authorite de sante (HAS) from France.

Buildings

Modern hospital buildings are designed to minimize the effort of medical personnel and the possibility of contamination while maximizing the efficiency of the whole system. Travel time for personnel within the hospital and the transportation of patients between units is facilitated and minimized. The building also should be built to accommodate heavy departments such as radiology and operating rooms while space for special wiring, plumbing, and waste disposal must be allowed for in the design.

However, the reality is that many hospitals, even those considered 'modern', are the product of continual and often badly managed growth over decades or even centuries, with utilitarian new sections added on as needs and finances dictate. As a result, Dutch architectural historian Cor Wagenaar has called many hospitals:

"... built catastrophes, anonymous institutional complexes run by vast bureaucracies, and totally unfit for the purpose they have been designed for ... They are hardly ever functional, and instead of making patients feel at home, they produce stress and anxiety."

Some newer hospital designs now try to reestablish design that takes the patient's psychological needs into account, such as providing for more air, better views, and more pleasant color schemes. These ideas hearken back to the late eighteenth century, when the concept of providing fresh air and access to the 'healing powers of nature' were first employed by hospital architects in improving their buildings.

Another major change which is still ongoing in many parts of the world is the change from a ward-based system (where patients are treated and accommodated in communal rooms, separated at best by movable partitions) to a room-based environment, where patients are accommodated in private rooms. The ward-based system has been described as very efficient, especially for the medical staff, but is considered to be more stressful for patients and detrimental to their privacy. A major constraint on providing all patients with their own rooms is however found in the higher cost of building and operating such a hospital, which causes some hospitals to charge for the privilege of private rooms.

Ninewells Hospital, Dundee, Scotland is currently one of the largest hospitals in the world, it also is one of the largest teaching hospitals. Ninewells also contains the first building in Britain designed by architect Frank Gehry, in conjunction with James F Stephen. The design was commissioned by Maggie's centres, the cancer support organisation, for their third centre at the hospital and was officially opened on 25 September 2003 by Bob Geldof. Also Ten million pounds has been spent redesigning and overhauling the paediatric department of the hospital and, in June 2006, it was opened officially under the name Tayside Children's Hospital.

3

Hospital Management

Hospitals are not merely profit making organizations, more over they have the responsibility of taking care of human health. Since they provide prestigious service, they have a higher value in the society. In order to maintain that value, hospitals must take utmost care in providing health care services. Proper co- ordination of resources like man, machine, money and material is required to maintain superior quality in services rendered. The Enterprise Resource Planning (ERP) tool called Hospital Information System developed by Dewsoft Solutions is an ideal package for integrating an entire healthcare organization. We serve you better, because we know you better.

Healthcare providers usually face the challenge of minimizing cost without compromising the quality of services. Since hospitals are concerned with the life of the patients, any small error can lead to an irrecoverable loss - we know these facts better than anyone else, that's why utmost care is taken in preparing this ERP solution for hospitals.

Organizational Structure of a Hospital

Objectives/Rationale

Every hospital, large or small, has an organizational structure that allows for the efficient management of departments.

Key Points

Power Point: Importance of Understanding Organizational Structure of Hospital;

A. facilitates the understanding of the hospital's chain of command.

B. shows which individual or department is accountable for each area of the hospital.

Complexity of Organizational Structure Depends on Size of Healthcare Facility; large acute care hospitals have complicated structures, whereas, the smaller institutions have a much simpler organizational structure;

Grouping of Hospital Departments Within the Organizational Structure;

A. Although each hospital department performs specific functions, departments are generally grouped according to similarity of duties.

B. Departments are also grouped together in order to promote efficiency of the healthcare facility.

C. Common organizational categories might include:

1. Administration Services (often referred to simply as "administration")
2. Informational Services
3. Therapeutic Services
4. Diagnostic Services
5. Support Services (sometimes referred to as "Environmental Services").

Administration Services—business people who "run" the hospital.

A. Hospital Administrators :

1. manage and oversee the operation of departments :
    a. oversee budgeting and finance
    b. establish hospital policies and procedures
    c. perform public relation duties
2. generally include: Hospital President, Vice Presidents, Executive Assistants, Department Heads.

Informational Services—documents and process information;

A. Admissions-often the public's first contact with hospital personnel :

1. checks patients into hospital :

a. responsibilities include: obtaining vital information (patient's full name, address, phone number, admitting doctor, admitting diagnosis, social security number, date of birth, all insurance information)

b. frequently, admissions will assign in-house patients their hospital room .

Therapeutic Services – provides treatment to patients;

A. includes the following departments:

1. Physical Therapy (PT) :

a. provide treatment to improve large-muscle mobility and prevent or limit permanent disability

b. treatments may include: exercise, massage, hydrotherapy, ultrasound, electrical stimulation, heat application.

2. Occupational Therapy (OT) :

a. goal of treatment is to help patient regain fine motor skills so that they can function independently at home and work

b. treatments might include: arts and crafts that help with hand-eye coordination, games and recreation to help patients develop balance and coordination, social activities to assist patient's with emotional health.

3. Speech/Language Pathology :

a. identify, evaluate, and treat patients with speech and language disorders

b. also help patients cope with problems created by speech impairments.

4. Respiratory Therapy (RT) :

a. treat patient's with heart and lung diseases

b. treatment might include: oxygen, medications, breathing exercises.

5. Medical Psychology :
   a. concerned with mental well-being of patients
   b. treatments might include: talk therapy, behavior modification, muscle relaxation, medications, group therapy, recreational therapies (art, music, dance).
6. Social Services :
   a. aid patients by referring them to community resources for living assistance (housing, medical, mental, financial)
   b. social worker specialties include: child welfare, geriatrics, family, correctional (jail).
7. Pharmacy :
   a. dispense medications per written orders of physician, dentists, etc.
   b. provide information on drugs and correct ways to use them
   c. ensure drug compatibility.
8. Dietary - responsible for helping patients maintain nutritionally sound diets :
9. Sports Medicine :
   a. provide rehabilitative services to athletes
   b. teaches proper nutrition
   c. prescribe exercises to increase strength and flexibility or correct weaknesses
   d. apply tape or padding to protect body parts
   e. administer first aid for sports injuries.
10. Nursing (RN, LVN, LPN) :
    a. provide care for patients as directed by physicians
    b. many nursing specialties include: nurse practitioner, labor and delivery nurse, neonatal nurse, emergency room nurse, nurse midwife, surgical nurse, nurse anesthetist

c. In some facilities, *Nursing* is a service in and of itself.

Diagnostic Services – determines cause(s) of illness or injury;

A. includes the following departments:
   1. Medical Laboratory (MT) - studies body tissues to determine abnormalities
   2. Imaging
      a. image body parts to determine lesions and abnormalities
      b. includes the following: Diagnostic Radiology, MRI, CT, Ultra Sound.
   3. Emergency Medicine - provides emergency diagnoses and treatment.

Support Services—provides support to entire hospital;

A. includes the following departments:
   1. Central Supply :
      a. in charge of ordering, receiving, stocking and distributing all equipment and supplies used by healthcare facility
      b. sterilize instruments or supplies
      c. clean and maintain hospital linen and patient gowns.
   2. Biomedical Technology :
      a. design and build biomedical equipment (engineers)
      b. diagnose and repair defective equipment (biomedical technicians)
      c. provide preventative maintenance to all hospital equipment (biomedical technicians)
      d. pilot use of medical equipment to other hospital employees (biomedical technicians).
   3. Housekeeping and Maintenance :
      a. maintain safe clean environment
      b. cleaners, electricians, carpenters, gardeners.

Hospitals: Organizational Structure and Quality Management

More than a decade ago, the WHO Health Promoting Hospitals (HPH) project was initiated in order to support hospitals towards placing greater emphasis on health promotion and disease prevention, rather than on diagnostic and curative services alone. The Health Promoting Hospitals strategy focuses on meeting the physical, mental and social needs of a growing number of chronically ill patients and the elderly; on meeting the needs of hospital staff, who are exposed to physical and psychological stress; and on meeting the needs of the public and the environment.

Twenty hospitals in eleven European countries participated in the European pilot project from 1993 to 1997. Since then, the International Network of Health Promoting Hospitals has steadily expanded and now covers 25 Member States, 36 national or regional networks and more than 700 partner hospitals.

But, what has been achieved with regard to the implementation of health promotion services at both hospital and network level? What is the scope of health promotion activities in hospitals and how can the principles laid out in the Ottawa Charter for Health Promotion be put into practice? Is there an evidence base for health promotion and has this facilitated the expansion of health promotion services in hospitals? Is health promotion a service anyway? How does health promotion relate to quality management? And how can we evaluate the quality of health promotion activities in hospitals? Health promotion: definition and concept

Health promotion measures focus on both individuals and on contextual factors that shape the actions of individuals with the aim to prevent and reduce ill health and improve wellbeing. Health in this context not only refers to the traditional, objective and biomedical view of the absence of infirmity or disease but to a holistic view that adds mental resources and social well-being to physical health. Health promotion goes beyond health education and disease prevention, in as far as it is based on the concept of salutogenesis and stresses the analysis and development of the health potential of individuals.

The scope of *disease prevention* has been defined in the Health Promotion Glossary as "measures not only to prevent the occurrence of disease, such as risk factor reduction, but also to arrest its progress and reduce its consequences once established". The same source defines the scope of *health education* as comprising "consciously constructed opportunities for learning involving some form of communication designed to improve health literacy, including improving knowledge and developing life skills which are conducive to individual and community health". Health promotion is defined as a broader concept in the WHO Ottawa Charter as "the process of enabling people to increase control over, and improve, their health".

In practice, these terms are frequently used complementarily and measures for the implementation may overlap; however, there are major conceptual differences with regard to the focus and impact of health promotion actions.

Whereas the medical approach is directed at physiological risk factors (e.g. high blood pressure, immunization status), the behavioural approach is directed at lifestyle factors (e.g. smoking, physical inactivity) and the socio-environmental approach is directed at general conditions (such as unemployment, low education or poverty). Health promotion consequently includes, but goes far beyond medical approaches directed at curing individuals.

Based on the notion of health as a positive concept, the Ottawa Charter put forward the idea that "health is created and lived by people within the settings of their everyday life; where they learn, work, play and love". This settings approach to health promotion, founded on the experience of community and organizational development, led to a number of initiatives such as Health Promoting Cities, Health Promoting Schools, and Health Promoting Hospitals, etc. in order to improve people's health where they spend most of their time: in organizations.

The settings approach acknowledges that behavioural changes are only possible and stable if they are integrated into everyday life and correspond with concurrent habits and existing cultures. Health Promotion interventions in organizations therefore not only have to address changing individuals but also underlying norms, rules and cultures. The Ottawa Charter identifies five priority action areas for health promotion:

- Build healthy public policy: health promotion policy combines diverse but complementary approaches, including legislation, fiscal measures, taxation and organization change. Health promotion policy requires the identification of obstacles to the adoption of healthy public policies in non-health sectors and the development of ways to remove them.
- Create supportive environments for health: the protection of the natural and build environments and the conservation of natural resources must be addressed in any health promotion strategy.
- Strengthen community action for health: Community development draws on existing human and material resources to enhance self-help and social support, and to develop flexible systems for strengthening public participation in, and direction of, health matters. This requires full and continuous access to information and learning opportunities for health, as well as funding support.
- Develop personal skills: Enabling people to learn (throughout life) to prepare themselves for all stages and to cope with chronic illness and injuries is essential. This has to be facilitated in school, home, work and community settings.
- Re-orient health services: the role of the health sector must move increasingly in a health promotion direction, beyond its responsibility for providing clinical and curative services. Reorientation of health services also requires stronger attention to health research, as well as changes in professional education and training.

The Impact of Health Services on Health

Many health professionals presume that health promotion has always been the core business of medicine in general and hospitals in particular. This view may be challenged for a variety of reasons.

Although the history goes back further, the first identifiable hospitals were built during the 12th century and were religious-oriented, cloister-affiliated institutions providing support to the poor, elderly, psychologically deviant and others in need. In the foreground were the accommodation, nourishment and the isolation of infectious diseases, not the treatment of disease.

Until the late 19th century hospitals were not a place where health was created, but rather a place to die. This changed with the development of the science of medicine, supported by utilitarian state philosophy and humanism. Since then, the potential of hospital care to improve health has made rapid improvements with the development of aseptic and antiseptic techniques, more effective anaesthesia, greater surgical knowledge and skills, trauma techniques, blood transfusion, coronary artery bypass surgery, effective pharmaceuticals, transplantation techniques and minimal invasive surgery . However, parallel to the advances in hospital procedures, questions have been raised with regard to the contribution of health care to the health of the population and the effectiveness of health care services. Various accounts have been made discarding the claims of health care for the reduction of infectious diseases, the significant decline in infant mortality, reductions in the major causes of death and resulting increase in life expectancy.

Although controversy is still continuing on details of his work, McKeown demonstrated compellingly how reductions in mortality in the United Kingdom, which were thought to be related to accomplishments of medical care, were in fact related to improvements in hygiene and nutrition. Another perspective was brought in by Ivan Illich and Rick Carlson who argued that medical care is more a cause of death, than of health. According to Illich, medicine has the potential to cause as much harm as good, as reflected in his concept of *iatrogenesis*. He strongly criticized the medical professions of their "sick-making powers" and contended that health care institutions performed the opposite of their original purpose. Carlson argued along the same lines and forecasted that the limited effectiveness of medicine will further decline in the future. Recently, these perspectives gained a lot of prominence with the report of the Institute of Medicine, "To err is human", which estimates that in the USA about 100,000 deaths in hospitals annually are due to medical errors.

A more operational perspective was brought in by the Avedis Donabedian and others who, being well aware of the limited population impact of health care, focused on strategies to improve the quality of health care services. Although major advances have been made with the outcomes movement and health technology assessment, the definition of quality as doing the right thing and doing it well, still raises fundamental questions and points to potential improvements in the provision of health care services.

The Health Promoting Hospitals network links the various perspectives above. It is driven by the strong perception that hospital services need to be more targeted towards the need of people, and not only to their organs or physiological parameters, in order to have a more substantial and lasting impact on health. At the same time the HPH philosophy is now based on strong evidence and methods to incorporate health promotion as a core principle in the organization. Quality strategies already applied in clinical settings and for the management of health care organizations are applicable to health promotion as well. Before addressing this issue further below, the following paragraphs provide the rationale for and concrete examples of health promotion services in hospitals.

Health Promotion Activities in Hospitals

Given the scope of possible health promotion interventions in hospitals, the WHO HPH movement focuses on four areas: promoting the health of patients, promoting the health of staff, changing the organization to a health promoting setting, and promoting the health of the community in the catchment area of the hospital. These four areas are reflected in the definition of a health promoting hospital:

"A *health promoting hospital* does not only provide high quality comprehensive medical and nursing services, but also develops a corporate identity that embraces the aims of health promotion, develops a health promoting organizational structure and culture, including active, participatory roles for patients and all members of staff, develops itself into a health promoting physical environment, and actively cooperates with its community".

There is a large scope and public health impact for offering health promotion strategies in health care settings. Hospitals consume between 40% and 70% of the national health care expenditure and typically employ about 1% to 3% of the working population. These working places, most of which are occupied by women, are characterized by certain physical, chemical, biological and psychosocial risk factors. Paradoxically, in hospitals – organizations that aim to restore health – the acknowledgement of factors that endanger the health of their staff is poorly developed. Health promotion programmes can improve the health of staff, reduce absenteeism rates, and improve productivity and quality

Health professionals in hospitals can also have a lasting impact on influencing the behaviour of patients and relatives, who are more responsive to health advice in situations of experienced ill-health. This is of particular importance for two reasons: firstly, the prevalence of chronic diseases (e.g. diabetes, cardiovascular diseases, cancer) is increasing in Europe and throughout the world; secondly, many hospital treatments today not only prevent premature death but improve the quality of life of patients. In order to maintain this quality, the patient's own behavior after discharge and effective support from relatives are important variables. Health Promotion Programmes can encourage healthy behavior, prevent readmission and maintain quality of life of patients.

Hospitals also typically produce high amounts of waste and hazardous substances. Introducing Health Promotion strategies in hospitals can help reduce the pollution of the environment and the cooperation with other institutions and professionals can help achieve the highest possible coordination of care. Furthermore, as research and teaching institutions hospital produce, accumulate and disseminate a lot of knowledge and they can have an impact on the local health structures and influence professional practice elsewhere.

Evolution of the International Network of Health Promoting Hospitals

In order to support the introduction of health promotion programmes in hospitals, the WHO Regional Office for Europe started the first international consultations in 1988. In the subsequent year, the WHO model project "Health and Hospital" was initiated with the hospital Rudolfstiftung in Vienna, Austria, as a partner institution. After this phase of consultation and experimenting the HPH movement went into its developmental phase, being marked by the initiation of the European Pilot Hospital Project by the WHO Regional Office for Europe in 1993. This phase, which lasted from 1993 to 1997, involved intensive monitoring of the development of projects in 20 partner hospitals from 11 European Countries.

Subsequent to the closing of this pilot phase, national and regional networks were developed and the network reached its consolidation phase. Since then, national and regional networks take an important role in encouraging the cooperation and exchange of experience between hospitals of a region or a country, including the identification of areas of common interest, the sharing of resources and the development of common evaluation systems. In addition, a thematic network exists, bringing together psychiatric hospitals and allowing the exchange of ideas and strategies in this particular field. The International Network of Health Promoting Hospitals acts as a network of networks linking all national/regional networks. It supports the exchange of ideas and strategies implemented in different cultures and health care systems, developing knowledge on strategic issues and enlarging the vision. As of May 2005, the International HPH Network comprises 25 Member States, 35 national and regional networks and more than 700 hospitals. As defined in the WHO Health Promotion Glossary, *"Health promotion* evaluation is an assessment of the extent to which health promotion actions achieve a *'valued' outcome"*. Assessment methods and outcomes differ in health promotion as compared to clinical medicine.

With the current focus of health system and hospital managers on outcomes, qualitative methods are frequently considered as offering only weak evidence. In fact, the longterm benefit of many health promotion interventions makes it necessary to distinguish between different levels of health promotion outcomes, beyond changes in clinical parameters and in health status. In the context of health promotion participation, partnership, empowerment and actions directed to the creation of supportive environments are also important aspects that need to be evaluated, and many proponents of health promotion indeed recommend different levels of analysis. Don Nutbeam suggests distinguishing outcomes according to health promotion outcomes, intermediate outcomes and health and social outcomes:

- *Health promotion outcomes* refer to modifications of personal, social and environmental factors to improve people's control over the determinants of health (e.g. health literacy, social influence and action, healthy public policy and organizational culture);
- *Intermediate outcomes* refer to changes in the determinants of health (e.g. lifestyles, access to health services, reduction of environmental risks);
- *Health and social outcomes* refer to subjective (self reported assessments such as Nottingham Health Profile, SF-36 or EUROQOL) and objective measures (weight, cholesterol level, blood pressure measurement, biochemical test, mortality) of changes in health and in social status (e.g. equity).

The HPH movement has provided many good examples of health promotion interventions that hospitals can carry out. Some of these interventions have been evaluated in the literature as being highly effective and cost-effective as described in the chapter on Evidence for Health Promotion in this volume. Some may discard the narrow view of health promotion activities that were evaluated using controlled designs, and argue that our understanding goes beyond these activities.

Assessment of Activities in Health Promoting Hospitals?

Currently, the quality of health promoting activities in the hospitals of the International HPH network is not systematically assessed. Hospitals becoming members of the International Network:

- endorse the fundamental principles and strategies for implementation of the Vienna Recommendations;
- belong to the National/Regional HPH Network in the countries where such networks exist (hospitals in countries without such networks apply directly to the international coordinating institution); and
- comply with the rules and regulations established at the international and national/regional levels.

Hospitals in the International Network further have to commit themselves to become a smoke-free hospital and to run three specific projects/activities addressing health issues of staff, patients, community, or improving organizational routines with a possible impact on health. A web-based database has been established to register projects and activities, providing information on key indicators of the hospital and on health promotion activities.

At the international level, attempts have been made to review and develop evaluation systems for health promotion. The Fourth and Fifth Annual Workshop of National and Regional Network Coordinators in 1998 and 1999 addressed the issue and concluded that so far, evaluations, if any, were mostly carried out at project level, only a few strategies of quality assurance were applied at network level and most coordinators experienced great problems in developing and applying evaluation schemes. There are different evaluation approaches at national and regional network levels, although none of them are well developed yet.

Among the most developed tools applied was the Hospital Accreditation Scheme that evolved from the Healthy Hospital Award in the United Kingdom. Hospitals were formally accredited as Health Promoting Hospital after application, standardized self-audit survey and external assessment to validate the survey and interview staff and patients.

A similar system was installed in the German system consisting of two peer-reviews from hospitals and one site-visit from a representative of the network to the applicant hospital. External assessors decided on the acceptance in the network. However, the German experience shows that, due to the financial implications, these visits are difficult to carry out. The German Network has also worked on adapting the excellence model of the European Foundation of Quality Management and the Balanced Scorecard for the systematic implementation of health promotion in the hospitals' organizational structure and culture. A report on the process of this work is also available in the present volume.

In 1994, the Polish Network started a self-assessment system to monitor the improvement of individual hospital performance; however, its application was not continued due to validity and reliability issues of the tool. The Danish Network decided in December 2000 to initiate the establishment of a set of standards; part of this work is also presented in this volume.

Other countries in the WHO European Region initiated in the past similar schemes consisting of site-visits, peer review, self-assessment, and surveys. Outside Europe, the Ministry of Health in Thailand conducted a survey comparing 17 Health Promoting Hospitals with 23 non-HPH. A questionnaire was designed and items were constructed for a self-assessment of HPH strategy implementation according to the following dimensions: a) Leadership and administration, b) Resource allocation and Human Resource development, c) Supportive environment, d) Health promotion for staff, e) Health promotion of patients and families, and f) Community health promotion. Many methodological issues need to be resolved before a valid comparison can be made; however, the survey contains many innovative ideas that may be elaborated in the future.

The Way Forward

Although a lot of progress has been made in the last decade, the idea of health promotion has only slowly been introduced to hospitals. Perhaps one of the main factors explaining this was the lack of clear strategies and tools for implementation.

There is now much better and stronger evidence for many health promotion interventions directed at patients, staff and the community. Likewise, tools have been developed to help health professionals to prioritize and implement health promotion.

Health Promoting Hospitals have committed themselves to integrate health promotion in daily activities and to follow the Vienna Recommendations, which advocate encouraging patient participation, involving all professionals, fostering patients' rights and promoting a healthy environment within hospitals. Thus, health promotion in hospitals includes interventions and actions. In order to ensure effective and efficient implementation of health promotion valid standards and guidelines are needed just as for other clinical activities. The evidence base for a wide range of interventions will be reviewed in the following sections.

Evidence-based Health Promotion in Hospitals

While "curative" medicine is delivered to symptomatic patients who seek health care, health promotion and preventive interventions will often attempt to modify individuals' lives, and this must be based on the highest level of randomized evidence "that our preventive manoeuvre will do more good than harm".

Practice guidelines are considered valid if "when followed, they lead to the health gains and the costs predicted for them", and they must be based on evidence from trials using valid methods. Evidence is usually categorized as:

- 1a: Evidence from meta-analysis of randomized controlled trials;
- 1b: Evidence from at least one randomized controlled trial;
- 2a: Evidence from at least one controlled study without randomization;
- 2b: Evidence from at least one other type of quasi-experimental study;
- 3: Evidence from descriptive studies, such as comparative studies, correlation studies and case-control studies;
- 4: Evidence from expert committee reports or opinions or clinical experience of respected authorities, or both.

Health promotion should be based on a high level of evidence, i.e. level 1a, 1b or 2a, whenever possible. Weaker evidence may be used for describing good clinical practice in health promotion in hospitals, but whenever category 1a to 2a is absent, it should be considered relevant to establish new evidence. Clinical trials in the spectre of health promotion must meet the same criteria for quality as other randomized trials. They are: Appropriateness of inclusion and exclusion criteria, concealment of allocation, blinding of patients and health professionals if possible, objective or blind method of data collection, valid or blind method of data analysis, completeness and length of follow up, appropriateness of outcome measures and statistical power of results.

The large group of qualitative studies are outside the evidence definition. They describe the opinions and feelings of selected persons, and they are based upon the specific interviewer's interpretation and competences, and the concrete context. They are important for an implementation process and may give rise to new hypothesis, but the results can seldom be generalized. Using both quantitative research and qualitative studies is a unique combination in exploring new areas for investigation and implementation.

Concepts Used

In public health, disease prevention is usually defined as a) primary disease prevention which prevents diseases from occurring, b) secondary prevention which detects disease at an early stage and prevents disease from developing, and c) tertiary prevention or rehabilitation which prevents aggravation or recurrence of disease and secures maintenance of functional level. Traditionally, hospitals primarily take care of tasks that relate to secondary or tertiary prevention whereas the primary sector and other social institutions take care of primary prevention. It is, however, increasingly recognized that also hospitals can play a significant role in primary prevention. When integrating health promotion in clinical activity it makes more sense to use a classification that distinguishes between patient pathways in ordinary clinical practice, staff and the community:

- Patients: General health promotion which should be offered to all patients and which addresses all patient pathways. Specific health promotion vis-a-vis defined patient groups, characterized through their belonging to certain diagnosis groups or otherwise.

- Staff: General health promotion aiming at a healthy and safe work environment. Training in the field of clinically related health promotion.
- Community: Cooperation with relevant structures and organizations.

General health promotion addresses general determinants of health and disease (including tobacco, alcohol, nutrition, physical activity and psychosocial issues). One example of this is lifestyle intervention, which involves activities aiming to influence individual behaviour (alcohol consumption, smoking etc.). Lifestyle intervention includes counselling, recommendations and empowering the patients to enhance their competence and their capability.

Specific health promotion addresses conditions that are significant for specific patient groups. Examples of this are the prevention of complications in diabetes patients, education of asthma patients, cardiac rehabilitation etc. An iinportant element in disease-related health promotion is strengthening the patient's ability to manage his/her condition.

Policy of Health Promotion in Hospitals

Hospitals are a special type of workplace with many employees that are exposed both physically and mentally in connection with their clinical tasks. In spite of work environment regulations, many exposures and risk situations cannot be avoided. Therefore it is necessary for hospitals to have a health promotion policy. On the basis of existing knowledge of the importance of lifestyle factors for treatment and prognosis, all hospitals should establish policy, counselling services, education and support for health promotion as an integrated part of the individual patient pathway as well as for the staff.

Effect of a health promotion policy in hospitals is based upon descriptive studies, exclusively, giving a low level of evidence.

Health Promotion for Hospital Staff

Those working in the health care sector can play an important role in promoting health, either through providing examples of what can be done to achieve a healthy environment or through using their authority to act as advocates for public health policies or in giving advice to individual patients or citizens.

Learning and teaching in methods used in health promotion and patient education should build on evidence. The individual lifestyle habits of health care staff, their attitudes and competencies influence the way they handle prevention issues.

Staff who are smokers generally underestimate the role of smoking as a risk factor, whereas non-smokers in some cases overestimate this risk factor. Thus smokers are less prone to advise patients on lifestyle issues in general and the same is true of staff that feel that they have too little training in this field. Staff who are smokers do not convey through their behaviour the health knowledge they are supposed to communicate to the patients; there is a cognitive disparity between their behaviour and their knowledge, i.e. staff either choose to stop smoking or ignore their knowledge to the detriment of advice for patients.

Interestingly, staff that stops smoking initiate more interventions among patients with improved effect. Special competences are another important way of improving the integration in the clinical daily life. The implementation rates are given for "spontaneous" motivational counselling in the emergency department, for the usual staff, and for specialist nurses in three successive periods, each including 100 patients. Specialized staff offer more systematic advice on smoking cessation than other staff.

Evidence for General Health Promotion

There is documentation for the effect of health promotion in relation to lifestyle factors.

Tobacco

Tobacco causes a wide range of diseases. Smoking causes 30% of all occurrences of ischaemic heart disease, explains 90% of lung cancer, 75% of chronic obstructive lung disease (smoker's lungs) and 6 % of hip fracture. Not only do diseases occur more frequently in smokers, they also occur at a younger age compared to non-smokers. And population studies show that there are twice as many admissions among smokers as among non-smokers. A great number of hospital admissions are related to patients' lifestyles. Tobacco related diseases cause 30% of all admissions in an ordinary medical ward. And in addition, tobacco plays an indirect role for many other admissions. Smoking also influences the outcome of treatment. It is well documented that medical treatment for hypertension, radiation treatment of cancers of the head and the neck, treatment of arteriosclerosis and wounds are much less effective in smokers than in non-smokers. Smoking influences the immune system and plays a role in the prolongation of hospital stay for patients with infections.

Patients' long term condition and prognosis are also influenced. There is documentation that patients who stop smoking following myocardial infarction diminish the risk of recurrence within the following two years by 50%.

Unplanned readmissions cause considerable expenditure for the health care sector. Smokers have almost twice as many readmissions as non-smokers. Studies show that the average rate of readmission amounts to between 16% and 27%; patients with ischaemic heart disease, smokers' lungs (COPD) and lung cancer have a particular high rate of readmissions.

Smoking cessation has a well-documented effect on symptoms and health. Many studies show a dose-response relation between exposure to tobacco (duration of smoking habit and amount smoked) and the occurrence of disease. Similarly, there is direct proportional relationship between how long a person has been smoke free and a reduced risk of disease. Recent studies document that even smoking cessation at the age of 65 has a positive effect on health and reduces morbidity, however, a reduction of the amount consumed plays no decisive role.

In short, documentation shows that smoking cessation:

- reduces or removes lung diseases such as coughing and expectorate in healthy smokers;
- normalizes future loss of lung function in patients with established chronic lung disease;

- reduces by half the risk of cancers after 5 years (former large scale smokers do, however, have an increased risk of lung cancer for the rest of their lives);
- leads to an immediate drop in the risk of cardiac and cerebral infarction;
- reduces by half the risk of another infarction and of death within the years following acute myocardial infarction;
- reduces the risk of arteriosclerosis and related diseases;
- reduces the risk of osteoporosis and resulting hip fracture;
- reduces the risk of giving birth to a premature infant if undertaken during the first 3 to 4 months of pregnancy;
- reduces the risk of late complications in patients with diabetes;
- improves the delayed healing process of wound and tissue healing.

The evidence is based upon descriptive studies of smoking and randomized clinical studies of stop smoking, giving a high level of evidence.

Alcohol

Large scale alcohol consumption adds to the risk of diseases such as pneumonia, infections, diarrhoea and malabsorption, dissemination of cancer, non-alcoholic liver disease, hypertension, poorly regulated diabetes, fluid and electrolyte imbalances. Patients with a high alcohol intake are more often admitted to hospital; about 20% of men and 10% of the women admitted to hospital consume alcohol in excess of internationally recommended limits.

Patients' alcohol consumption also influences the outcome of treatment and care. The mechanisms include reduced immune function, sub clinical or clinical cardiac dysfunction, haemostatic imbalance, delayed healing of wound and slow tissue and bone turnover, myopathy, and increased stress-response; all contribute to prolongation of hospital stay for the patients.

There is evidence that cessation and to some degree reduction of alcohol consumption leads to:

- fewer admissions with alcohol related disorders such as cirrhosis of the liver and Pancreatitis;
- fewer admissions due to poisoning, alcoholism and alcohol psychosis;
- fewer infections (especially pneumonia and tuberculosis);
- improved wound and bone healing;
- improved heart function and blood pressure;
- improved outcome for several non-alcoholic diseases (among other effects).

The evidence is based upon descriptive studies of alcohol intake and randomized clinical studies of stop drinking as well as randomized studies of voluntary excessive alcohol intake, giving a high level of evidence.

Physical Activity

Lack of physical activity is associated with increased occurrence of type 2 diabetes, overweight, high blood fat levels, hypertension and development of metabolic syndrome.

There is evidence that regular physical activity:

- reduces the risk of developing cardiovascular disease in general and ischaemic heart disease in particular;
- reduces the risk of developing type 2 diabetes;
- reduces mortality in middle-aged and elderly persons of both sexes;
- strengthens the development of bone density, restrains age related drop in bone mineral content and prevents the development of osteoporosis;
- prevents hypertension and reduces hypertension;
- prevents overweight;
- prevents depression, reduces tension and increases self-respect;
- prevents loss of muscle mass in elderly patients and reduces the risk of falls.

Physical training is an important element in several rehabilitation programmes, e.g. cardiac rehabilitation, rehabilitation of chronic obstructive lung disease, surgical rehabilitation, psychiatric rehabilitation etc.

Physical training for patients with myocardial infarction reduces the risk of another infarction by 25% in the first three years. Training is also an important element in mobilization of patients with rheumatoid arthritis and patients with arthritis, and studies have shown that exercise in the form of walks may put off the time of surgical intervention for patients who are waiting for knee or hip replacement.

The evidence is based upon descriptive studies of physical activity and randomized clinical studies, giving a high level of evidence.

Nutrition

In the European population, overweight is the most common health problem. The increasing prevalence of overweight leads to a growing number of persons with diabetes, cardiovascular disease, strain injury and hormone related cancers. However, a problem encountered by hospitals is under-nourishment. Studies show that almost 30 % of hospital patients are undernourished on admission. At the same time, studies show that patients' food intake during hospital stay often amounts to only 60% of their actual needs.

There is documentation that undernourished patients have increased morbidity and mortality than well-nourished patients. At the same time, there is documentation that systematic screening of nutrition status and proper nutritional therapy during admission reduce the risk of wound infection and lead to shorter hospital stay and contribute to more rapid convalescence. There is evidence that nutritional interventions in relation to undernourished patients:

- improve lung functions and walking distance in patients with chronic lung disease;
- increase weight and muscle mass in patients with cancer;
- increase physical activity and reduces mortality in geriatric patients;
- reduce mortality in patients with acute renal failure.

The evidence is based upon several randomized clinical studies, giving a high level of evidence.

Recommendations with Regard to Hospital Tasks

There is international consensus that patients should be given recommendations, guidance and support with regard to health promotion in hospitals. Health promotion secures that risk conditions are identified and that the patient has knowledge of the significance of these conditions, recommendations for changes and active support for carrying out these changes. Evidence exists for the following interventions, which should be implemented in general hospital practice:

Tobacco

- identification of smokers and establishing a thorough tobacco history;
- oral and written information to patients on damaging effects and health benefits, and the possibility of smoking cessation;
- advice and recommendations with regard to cessation;
- establishing smoking cessation services or integration of smoking cessation counselling as part of treatment.

Alcohol

- identification of patients with harmful and dependent alcohol consumption according to ICD-10 criteria;
- oral and written information to patients on damaging effects and health benefits and the possibilities of assistance to stop or reducing consumption;
- recommendations for large scale consumers to stop or reduce consumption;
- offering brief interventions (for harmful intake) or referral to alcohol unit (for dependent intake).

Physical Activity

- identification of patients with a need for counselling on physical activity;

- counselling on exercise in accordance with international guidelines, and followup and counselling in connection with subsequent contacts with the department;
- establishing systematic training programmes for relevant patients (heart and lung patients, diabetes, surgery, psychiatry, overweight and underweight).

Nutrition

- identification of undernourished patients and patients at risk of undernourishment;
- initiation of relevant nutrition treatment and continued observation of body weight and food intake throughout the patient's stay in hospital;
- communication of information on discharge (to own doctor, home care, general practitioner);
- identification of overweight patients and screening for diabetes and other complications;
- counselling on diet and physical training;
- establishing of systematic training programmes for relevant patients;
- secure follow up in the primary health care sector.

Systematic Intervention and Patient Education

The aim of health counselling is to support the individual's process of change with regard to lifestyle. Health counselling is based on theories of behavioural change. The theories describe the phases and processes that people go through when they change behaviour. The model describes behavioural change as a circular process. Most people go through the process several times before they finally change behaviour. Health counselling consists of a dialogue with the patient and is based on:

- the patient's knowledge of the influence of tobacco and alcohol on health and the significance of cessation/ reduction for disease, treatment and health;
- the patient's ideas, emotions and attitudes with regard to the consumption under consideration;

- the patient's previous experiences when trying to change habits;
- recognition of the patient's emotions with regard to consumption;
- acceptance of the patient's choice with regard to consumption and;
- setting realistic goals for the outcome of the interview that correspond to the phase of change that the patient is going through.

There is evidence that health counselling may be used to motivate lifestyle changes. Since 1996, the Bispebjerg Hospital (Copenhagen, Denmark) has been trying to develop systematic intervention with regard to alcohol and tobacco, which includes health counselling for all patients including outpatients, elective patients, day patients and acutely admitted patients.

Evidence for Specific Prevention

Specific prevention concerns prevention activities addressing specific groups of patients. Patient education and rehabilitation programmes are examples of this. Rehabilitation programmes that aim to support the individual's own ability to manage disease are thus part of the clinical guidelines for several patient groups, not as a supplementary aspect, but as part of treatment. The various education and rehabilitation programmes include common elements, e.g. counselling on smoking cessation, stopping or reducing alcohol intake, physical activity, nutrition, psychosocial support, patient education and optimizing the medical (or surgical or psychiatric) treatment.

Heart Patients

Ischaemic heart disease is one of the biggest disease groups in the hospital sector and is the source of large, and ever increasing, pressure of demand on the health care sector altogether. Formerly rehabilitation of heart patients primarily concerned physical training, but against the background of the scientific results achieved over the past 10 to 15 years, the concept of heart rehabilitation has been extended to cover the following elements:

- physical training;
- lifestyle intervention and risk factor control: support to change of eating habits, smoking cessation, alcohol reduction, moderate physical training and preventive medical treatment;
- patient education;
- psychosocial care;
- medical treatment of symptoms;
- systematic control and follow up.

Results from international, controlled studies show evidence that heart rehabilitation may provide significant health outcomes in the form of:

- reduction of the number of admissions, both readmissions and overall cardiac admissions;
- maintenance of the patient's functional level;
- improvement of the patient's health related quality of life;
- improvement of overall risk factor control through lifestyle change and enhanced medical compliance.

There is a high level of evidence for the value of cardiac rehabilitation.

Chronic Lung Patients

Chronic obstructive lung disease (COPD) is a frequently occurring disease and is the cause of 20 to 25 % of admissions to medical departments in Europe. COPD is one of the five most resource demanding diseases in Denmark. Over the past 20 years many different lung rehabilitation programmes have been developed and tested, and there is now documentation that these programmes lead to:

- alleviation of breathing difficulty;
- increase in the distance that the patient is able to walk;
- improved physical capacity;
- improved functional level in everyday life;
- improved quality of life;

- improved ability to cope with disease and aggravation of disease;
- fewer admissions.

It is still not clear what the optimum structure, content and duration of COPD rehabilitation programmes is, however, there is agreement that as a minimum the following elements should be included:

- smoking cessation assistance;
- physical training/training in the home;
- physiotherapy;
- nutritional counselling;
- psychosocial support;
- patient education.

There is a moderate to high level of evidence for the value of rehabilitation after lung disease.

Asthma Patients

Asthma is a widespread disease, which occurs in about 5% of the adult population and in 5 to 10% of school children in most European countries. Over the past 30 to 40 years, a large number of randomized studies have been carried out in order to throw light on the effect of various education programmes. The programmes have been tested both in the hospital sector and in general practice. The resulting evidence has been summarized in several reviews and a Cochrane study, which conclude that there is documentation that patients who take part in asthma education programmes focusing on the training of skills achieve considerable effects, such as:

- fewer admissions;
- less absence from work;
- fewer asthma attacks at night;
- improvement of the patient's general capacity;
- improved medical compliance;
- improved quality of life.

It is still not clear what the optimum structure, content and duration of education programmes for asthma patients is. Usually programmes cover 4 to 5 lessons in the course of a couple of weeks.

There is a high level of evidence for the value of rehabilitation among asthma patients.

Diabetes Patients

Type 1-diabetes occurs in all age groups. Less is known about the occurrence of type 2- diabetes than about type 1-diabetes. The occurrence of type 2-diabetes is increasing rapidly and because of the increase in overweight/obesity it is seen in younger and younger persons. With regard to both types of diabetes the most significant health risk is development of late complications (risk of cardiovascular disease increased 3 to 5 times) and occurrence of diabetic eye disease, renal disorder and nervous disorder (retinopathy, nephropathy and neuropathy).

A number of randomized and controlled studies have been carried out with regard to both type 1 and type 2 diabetes. These studies all show that interventions with regard to one or several risk factors that can lead to late complications are effective .

Interventions should address:

- near normalization of blood sugar;
- near normalization of blood pressure and blood fat levels;
- smoking cessation;
- psychosocial support;
- counselling on nutrition, including alcohol, and physical activity.

There is a high level of evidence for the value of diabetic rehabilitation.

Osteoporosis Patients

There is an increase in the prevalence of osteoporosis in the western world, among other things because of an increase in the number of elderly persons. The risk of osteoporosis-related fractures increases considerably with age and is especially frequent in women. The three most frequent osteoporosis-related fractures occur in different age groups. Fracture in or near the wrist increases markedly from the age of 55, back problems from the age of 65, and fracture in or around the hip from the age of 75.

There is evidence that increased calcium intake in childhood may increase bone mineral content. There is no agreement as to whether women may benefit from calcium intake after the menopause.

But there are studies that indicate that calcium intake along with vitamin D, reduce the number of fractures in elderly men and women. Physical activity and an active lifestyle increase bone mineral content along with enhanced muscle strength and muscle coordination, which contributes to reduction of the risk of fractures. Smoking increases the risk of osteoporosis in women because female smokers have an earlier menopause than non-smokers and enhanced oestradiol metabolism. In the same way alcohol abuse in men constitutes a significant risk factor for the development of osteoporosis because of poor nutrition and reduced testosterone production.

Thus primary prevention should address:

- smoking cessation;
- reduction or cessation of alcohol consumption;
- motivation for physical activity.

Furthermore there is evidence that hip protectors reduce the number of fractures by 67% among elderly persons in rest homes. Thus hip protectors are an important element of the prevention programmes for frail elderly persons who are prone to falls and osteoporosis.

There is a low to moderate high level of evidence for rehabilitation among these patients.

Patients with Cancer

A reduction of the occurrence of cancer is a primary goal in health care plans in most countries whereas rehabilitation of cancer patients has not been considered equally. It is estimated that two thirds of newly diagnosed cancer patients need rehabilitation services.

It is necessary to initiate further knowledge in this area, however interventions should address:

- psychosocial support and counselling;
- physical training/relaxation;
- nutrition guidance;
- smoking cessation;
- sexual problems;
- communication of knowledge to patients and relatives.

There is a low level of evidence for cancer rehabilitation.

Stroke

Stroke is a serious condition in so far as 40% of the patients die during the first year after onset of the disease, and many patients are not able to return to their own homes.

Many factors increase the risk of stroke: smoking, alcohol abuse, lack of physical activity, increased blood fat levels, hypertension, diabetes, irregular heartbeat. The risk increases with age. There is evidence that patients participating in rehabilitation in the form of comprehensive interdisciplinary treatment through all the phases of the disease may achieve:

- a reduction of mortality of 25%-50%;
- a reduced need for residential homes of 40%;
- improved functional level.

Furthermore prevention includes counselling on smoking cessation, stop drinking or reduction of alcohol consumption, regulation of blood fat levels, optimization of blood pressure and heart function as well as anticoagulant therapy. Thus, it is recommended that patients with stroke are admitted to special stroke units where rehabilitation may be initiated already in the acute phase.

There is a high level of evidence for rehabilitation after apoplexy.

Patients with Psychiatric Disorders

A large proportion of psychiatric patients is smokers or have other substance abuse problems. Treatment with psychoactive medicine leads to considerable weight gain in many patients and therefore there is a need for intervention with regard to nutrition and physical activity. Physical activity in psychiatric patients has a documented positive effect on the course of treatment. Thus, prevention should be integrated in psychiatric patient pathways in the same way as in somatic pathways.

Work has been carried out concerning documentation and evaluation of various ways of organizing treatment, e.g. in the form of Assertive Community Treatment teams. There is evidence that Assertive Community Treatment Teams that address patients with a large use of inpatient days may reduce the cost of hospital treatment, increase the number who are in contact with the treatment system, and improve user satisfaction among patients and relatives. There is also a positive effect with regard to a number of social parameters, e.g. homelessness or not having an independent home. It is recommended that outreach psychosis teams be introduced generally for the treatment of patients with long-term psychotic disorders.

There is a high to moderate level of evidence for psychiatric rehabilitation.

Surgical Patients

A varying number of patients that undergo surgical intervention suffer from long-term and complicated conditions. The development of complications can be related to the diagnosis and the spread of the disease, type of intervention and the organization, i.e. staff competence, use of clinical guidelines etc. In recent years, we have acquired new knowledge on the significance of the patient's general lifestyle habits with regard to tobacco, alcohol, nutrition and exercise in connection with intervention. There is now evidence that targeted prevention initiatives can reduce the number of complications.

The significance of increased risk of complications due to the above mentioned factors should form part of overall indications for surgery. As in the case of intervention with regard to medical patients with chronic disorders, qualitative intervention should comprise seven elements, i.e. tobacco, alcohol, physical activity, nutrition, psychosocial support, medical (including surgical and anaesthetic) optimization and patient education.

Against the backdrop of available evidence, the National Board of Health has established general recommendations for intervention with regard to tobacco and alcohol in connection with surgical intervention. Early mobilization and nutrition have been described as significant elements of the postoperative phase.

Smoking

Altogether smokers have three times as many complications in the form of poor healing of wounds and other tissue and heart and lung complications in connection with surgical intervention compared to non-smokers.

Alcohol

Excessive alcohol consumption is linked to increased surgical risk, which increases with consumption so that there are three times as many complications in patients who consume five or more units per day. Complications are due to alcohol-induced organ damage that is reversible to a wide extent if no alcohol is consumed.

Nutrition

There is evidence that nutritional intervention for undernourished patients reduces complications in connection with surgical intervention by 10% and reduces the frequency of infection and increases muscle strength in surgical patients.

There is also evidence that resumption of food intake immediately after intervention considerably reduces complications.

Physical Activity

Early mobilization and increased physical activity following surgery has turned out to be significant and is part of a new overall concept for rehabilitation in connection with surgery. The intervention reduces weight loss and the fatigue often seen after surgery.

Preventive intervention that should be offered systematically:

- identification of risk factors;

- dialogue with the patient to clarify the role of these factors and the patients' own responsibility and options for influencing their own situation;
- evidence-based offer of intervention and follow up.

Intervention with regard to surgical patients is supported by the high motivation for changes in lifestyle prior to surgery, as measured by surprisingly high compliance. Patient information should include the high postoperative morbidity related to lifestyle factors, and the evidence based programme should be offered in due time before surgery.

The level of evidence is high to moderate with regard to prevention and rehabilitation in relation to surgery.

Empowerment of Patients for Health Promoting Self Care/ Self Maintenance/ Self Reproduction in the Hospital

Even if patients are not only understood as the object of treatment but also as coproducers of their health outcomes, we have to take into account that they can only fulfil their patient role in relation to the trinity of body, psyche, social status). Depending on their condition, the patient's contribution to co-production ranges selfcare of the patient, over professionally supported care to intensive care (heart/lung machine). Following the four criteria of the complex concept of health gain, reproduction concerns all three dimensions of health – the physical (e.g. adequate nutrition), the mental (e.g. enough privacy in the hospital), and the social (e.g. possibilities for contacts with relatives, patient support).

In order to avoid hospitalization as far as possible, it should be made a principle to allow for as much selfcare as possible, and to provide as much professional care as necessary. To make selfcare possible under the difficult conditions of partly severely ill individuals outside their usual household environment, and subjected to the bureaucratic imperatives of the hospital organization, professional care has to be as empowering as possible, and needs to take into account cultural differences of patients. Empowerment again includes physical, mental and social dimensions, knowledge, skills and motivations. This again can be seen as the specific contribution of health promotion.

The effects of this strategy have not been systematically researched, but examples of interventions that have been successfully implemented in specific hospitals are:

- visiting and lay support services to support the psychosocial needs of patients;
- patient information about general hospital features (e.g. where to find what; visiting hours) at hospital admission;
- offers and options to encourage patient activities and patient self-responsibility (e.g. exercise, culture activities, patient libraries, discussions, patient internet cafe);
- provide psychological assistance to cope with stress or anxieties related to the hospital stay or to the patient's disease (e.g. cancer).

Empowerment of Patients for Health Promoting Participation / Co-production in Treatment and Care

The core task of the modern acute care hospital is to offer diagnostic and therapeutic services for incidents of acute illness (of a rather severe type or with the need / opportunity for technical diagnostics and treatment) as well as acute episodes of chronic disease – for inpatients and outpatients.

The second health promotion strategy relates to the long and changing tradition of quality assurance and quality improvement of core tasks – starting with the education of professionals, and in the last 20 years switching towards developing processes and structures of organizations and larger systems. How can health promotion contribute to the quality improvement of core processes in hospitals?

The concept of empowerment stresses the necessity that individuals take control over their health – which means in the context of the hospital that patients are not only seen as objects of interventions but also as co-producers of these interventions – an idea that fits well with other traditions of analysing services as co-produced. As the co-producer has to actively contribute to the process, he / she has to be actively empowered for making this contribution. This sort of empowerment cannot be achieved by the clinical/technical interventions themselves, but by communicative/

educative interventions. Medicine has to open itself towards education. Education refers to the transfer of knowledge (data, information), training of skills and enhancement of motivation.

The concept of health gain defines the relevant output of the hospital interventions in a more complex way: clinical outcome + quality of life + patient satisfaction + health literacy. These outcomes refer to all three aspects of health: physical, mental and social. The treatment process itself has to become more complex. The focus stays on effective treatment, but in order to optimize health gain, aspects of disease prevention, health protection and health development have to get due attention within treatment (systematically avoid risks, use opportunities to build health resources – biological, mental, social).

A practical example for empowering patients for co-production would be diagnosisand treatment related patient information, training and counselling (e.g. by informing patients about how they can contribute to the recuperation process; by describing alternatives and side effects), in order to enable patients to participate in the diagnostic process (e.g. by providing all information needed); participate in treatment-related decision-making; participate in treatment and care processes (e.g. by complying with the prescriptions).

There is clear evidence that this type of patient empowerment can, e.g. for surgical patients, reduce post-surgical complications, and can speed up recovery. Development of the Hospital into a supportive, health promoting and empowering setting for patients.

The hospital does not only consist of service processes, but also of a context within which the services are provided. Just like the services produce (health) outputs / outcomes, the context / situation / setting has impacts that are relevant for health.

There are impacts of the material setting (hospital infections, quality of air, temperature, sick building syndrome etc.) and also impacts of the hospital as a social setting with its organizational structure and culture, that influence opportunities for coproduction and selfcare of patients and of course the professional treatment and care for patients.

What is the contribution of HP for settings development? Health promotion pays specific attention to supportive environments – physical as well as social, and enlarges the focus on results from clinical outcomes also to other dimensions of health gain.

New Health Promotion Services for Hospital Patients

Empowerment of Patients for Health Promoting Management of Chronic Illness

Expert interventions in hospitals provide in general only a turning point in disease processes, and a basis for recuperation or the successful management of chronic illness. The main part of recuperation or of the day-to-day illness management (prevention of aggravation, negative long-term effects, social consequences etc.) has to be performed primarily by the patients themselves – with specific professional support by the hospital, specialized services, the family doctor or other health care services and lay support. This phase of the illness career lasts much longer and is out of direct control of the hospital, but is crucial for the outcome of regaining health and quality of life.

Professional support for this phase is in its core educative: primarily information, consultation, and training.

Hospitals have to take this mid-range perspective on the illness career into account by either providing necessary disease specific support by themselves or by referring patients to other, specialized providers in the health care system. The more complex and the more rare the disease and its treatment gets, the more likely it remains a task of the hospital itself, but this of course requires adequate legal and financial regulation which allows to provide these services systematically. Within the International HPH network, there are many examples of effective interventions of this type of services, e.g. diabetes training, COPD training.

Empowerment of Patients for Health Promoting Lifestyle Development

The health gain of hospital interventions can be even further increased when taking on a more long term perspective. Future health can be improved by lifestyle changes – thus reducing disease-related risks and developing positive health potentials and resources. It is primarily educative services (information, consultation, training) that can be utilized to influence individual lifestyles. These types of services can be offered by different providers, e.g. other providers in health care, social services and adult education.

Hospitals are in a good position to offer such services, having already developed a relationship with patients in a crisis situation, being centres of knowledge and having a high prestige in the area of health. Health education can become a module in a package of educational communication, using the opportunity of the relationship and the time in the hospital. Investments in this direction would help to develop hospitals into genuine health centres.

4

Laboratory Safety in Hospital Management

Medical Laboratory

A medical laboratory or clinical laboratory is a laboratory where tests are done on clinical specimens in order to get information about the health of a patient as pertaining to the diagnosis, treatment, and prevention of disease.

Departments

Laboratory medicine is generally divided into four sections, and each of which is further divided into a number of units. These four sections are:

- Anatomic Pathology: units are included here, namely histopathology, cytopathology, and electron microscopy. Academically, each unit is studied alone in one course. Other courses pertaining to this section include anatomy, physiology, histology, pathology, and pathophysiology.
- Clinical Microbiology: This is the largest section in laboratory medicine; as it encompasses five different sciences (units). These include bacteriology, virology, parasitology, immunology, and mycology.
- Clinical Biochemistry: Units under this busy section are instrumental analysis, enzymology, toxicology and endocrinology.
- Hematology: This busy, section consists of three units, which are coagulation and blood bank and hematology.

Genetics is also studied along with a subspecialty known as cytogenetics. Distribution of clinical laboratories in health institutions varies greatly from one place to another. Take for example microbiology, some health facilities have a single laboratory for microbiology, while others have a separate lab for each unit, with nothing called a "microbiology" lab. Here's a detailed breakdown of the responsibilities of each unit:

- Microbiology receives almost any clinical specimen, including swabs, feces, urine, blood, sputum, cerebrospinal fluid, synovial fluid, as well as possible infected tissue. The work here is mainly concerned with cultures, to look for suspected pathogens which, if found, are further identified based on biochemical tests. Also, sensitivity testing is carried out to determine whether the pathogen is sensitive or resistant to a suggested medicine. Results are reported with the identified organism(s) and the type and amount of drug(s) that should be prescribed for the patient.
- Parasitology is a microbiology unit that investigates parasites. The most frequently encountered specimen here is faeces. However, blood, urine, sputum, and other samples may also contain parasites.
- Virology is concerned with identification of viruses in specimens such as blood, urine, and cerebrospinal fluid.
- Hematology works with whole blood to do full blood counts, and blood films as well as many other specialised tests.
- Coagulation requires citrated blood samples to analyze blood clotting times and coagulation factors.
- Clinical Biochemistry usually receives serum or plasma. They test the serum for chemicals present in blood. These include a wide array of substances, such as lipids, blood sugar, enzymes, and hormones.
- Toxicology mainly tests for pharmaceutical and recreational drugs. Urine and blood samples are submitted to this lab.

- Immunology/Serology uses the concept of antigen-antibody interaction as a diagnostic tool. Compatibility of transplanted organs is also determined.
- Immunohaematology, or Blood bank determines blood groups, and performs compatibility testing on blood donors and recipients. It also prepares blood components, derivatives, and products for transfusion.
- Urinalysis tests urine for many analytes. Some health care providers have a urinalysis laboratory, while others don't. Instead, each component of the urinalysis is performed at the corresponding unit. If measuring urine chemicals is required, the specimen is processed in the clinical biochemistry lab, but if cell studies are indicated, the specimen should be submitted to the cytopathology lab, and so on.
- Histopathology processes solid tissue removed from the body (biopsies) for evaluation at the microscopic level.
- Cytopathology examines smears of cells from all over the body (such as from the cervix) for evidence of inflammation, cancer, and other conditions.
- Electron microscopy prepares specimens and takes micrographs of very fine details by means of TEM and SEM.
- Genetics mainly performs DNA analysis.
- Cytogenetics involves using blood and other cells to get a karyotype. This can be helpful in prenatal diagnosis (e.g. Down's syndrome) as well as in cancer (some cancers have abnormal chromosomes).
- Surgical pathology examines organs, limbs, tumors, fetuses, and other tissues biopsied in surgery such as breast mastectomys.

Medical Laboratory Staff

The following is the hierarchy of the clinical laboratory staff from highest authority to lowest:

- Medical Director

- Pathologist, Clinical Biologist, Microbiologist, Biochemist,
- Resident in Pathology or Clinical Biology
- Pathologist Assistant, Microbiologist Assistant, Medical Biochemist Assistant,
- Laboratory Manager,
- Department Supervisor,
- Chief/Lead Technologist,
- Cytotechnologist, Medical Laboratory Scientist, Histotechnologist,
- Medical Laboratory Technician, Histotechnician
- Medical Laboratory Assistant (Lab Aide),
- Phlebotomist,
- Transcriptionist,
- Specimen processor, Secretary).

Some of these titles don't exist in some countries. Sometimes technologists and technicians do the same work. In France, clinical biologists may also be Medical director and laboratory manager.

Types of Laboratory

In many countries, there are two main types of labs that process the majority of medical specimens. Hospital laboratories are attached to a hospital, and perform tests on patients. Private (or community) laboratories receive samples from general practitioners, insurance companies, and other health clinics for analysis. These can also be called reference laboratories where more unusual and obscure tests are performed. For extremely specialised tests, samples may go to a research laboratory. A lot of samples are sent between different labs for uncommon tests. It is more cost effective if a particular laboratory specializes in a rare test, receiving specimens (and money) from other labs, while sending away tests it cannot do.

In many countries there are mainly three types of Medical Laboratories as per the types of investigations carried out. Clinical Pathology. Clinical Microbiology & Clinical Biochemistry laboratories. Clinical Pathology: Haematology, Histopathology,

Cytology, Routine Pathology. Clinical Microbiology: Bacteriology, Mycobacteriology, Virology, Mycology, Parasitology, Immunology, Serology. Clinical Biochemistry: Biochemical analysis, Hormonal assays etc. Blood Banks:- Blood bank is a separate body. Its laboratory need Microbiological analysis for infectious diseases that may be found in blood. Pathology to observe Blood grouping, Haematology & cross matching reactions. It also involves PRO department for the communication & contact for blood donations etc..

Specimen Processing and Work Flow

Sample processing will usually start with a set of samples and a request form.

Typically a set of vacutainer tubes containing blood, or any other specimen, will arrive to the laboratory in a small plastic bag, along with the form.

The form and the specimens are given a laboratory number. The specimens will usually all receive the same number, often as a sticker that can be placed on the tubes and form. This label has a barcode that can be scanned by automated analyzers and test requests uploaded from the LIS. Entry of requests onto a laboratory management system involves typing, or scanning (where barcodes are used) in the laboratory number, and entering the patient identification, as well as any tests requested. This allows laboratory machines, computers and staff to know what tests are pending, and also gives a place (such as a hospital department, doctor or other customer) for results to go.

For biochemistry samples, blood is usually centrifuged and serum is separated. If the serum needs to go on more than one machine, it can be divided into separate tubes.

Many specimens end up in one or more sophisticated automated analysers, that process a fraction of the sample and return one or more "results". Some laboratories use robotic sample handlers (Laboratory automation) to optimize the workflow and reduce contamination risk and sample handling of the staff.

The work flow in a lab is usually heavy from 2:00 am to 10:00 am. Nurses and doctors generally have their patients tested at least once a day with general complete blood counts and chemistry profiles. These orders are then drawn during a morning run by phlebotomists for results to be available in the patient's charts for the attending physicians to consult during their morning rounds. Another busy time for the lab is after 3:00 pm when private practice physician offices are closing. Couriers will pick up specimens that have been drawn throughout the day and deliver them to the lab. Also, couriers will stop at outpatient drawing centres and pick up specimens. These specimens will be processed in the evening and overnight to ensure results will be available the following day.

Laboratory Informatics

Laboratories today are held together by a system of software programs and computers that exchange data about patients, test requests, and test results known as a Laboratory information system or LIS. The LIS is interfaced with the hospital information system.

This system enables hospitals and labs to order the correct test requests for each patient, keep track of individual patient or specimen histories, and help guarantee a better quality of results as well as printing hard copies of the results for patient charts and doctors to check.

Result Analysis, Validation and Interpretation

According to ISO 15189 norm, all pathological results must be verified by a competent professional. In some countries staff like clinical scientists do the majority of this work inside the laboratory with abnormal results referred to the relevant pathologist. In others, only medical staff (pathologist or clinical biologist) is concerned by this phase. It can be assisted by some software in order to validate normal or non modified results. Medical staff are sometimes also required in order to explain pathology results to physicians. For a simple result given by phone or for a technical problem it's a medical technologist explaining it to a registered nurse.

Departments in some countries are exclusively directed by a specialized Pathologist, in others a consultant, medical or non-medical, may be the Head of Department. Clinical Scientists have the right to interpret and discuss pathology results in their discipline in many countries, in Europe they are qualified to at least Masters level, may have a PhD and can have an exit qualification equivalent to medical staff e.g. FRC Path in the UK. In France only medical staff (Pharm.D. and M.D. specialized in Anatomical pathology or Clinical biology) can discuss pathological results, clinical scientists are not considered as a part of medical staff.

Scandal in the Clinical lab Industry

As medical technology advanced doctors were able to get more and more tests done in shorter and shorter amounts of time. Where in the past a doctor might order a potassium and glucose and it would take hours for the results, now a doctor can order a full chemistry panel of 20 or more different analytes and get the results in under an hour. The results are also much more accurate and reliable now than in the past. Thus, into the 1970s and 1980s the lab became a source of profit within the hospital structure.

Some commercial labs began taking illegal and nefarious actions to increase their income. These practices included medicare and medicaid fraud by performing and billing for tests that the ordering physician never ordered, paying kickbacks to private doctor offices for sending their specimens to these reference labs, and other complicated criminal activity. These kickbacks included donuts, free computers, fax machines, and more. These events culminated mostly in the mid-1990s with the SmithKline Beecham Clinical Laboratory (SBCL) scandal. It is believed SBCL paid at least $325 million in penalties and the industry as a whole paid over $1 billion to insurance and government agencies that were defrauded. Ever since this time, the lab has become a source of expense and loss in the hospital budget (commercial labs have nothing to do with hospitals) and lab medicine's reputation was given a black eye. Now many labs have a compliance officer with mandatory annual meetings about compliance for all employees.

Medical Laboratory Accreditation

Credibility of medical laboratories is paramount to the health and safety of the patients relying on the testing services provided by these labs. The international standard in use today for the accreditation of medical laboratories is ISO 15189 - Medical laboratories - particular requirements for quality and competence.

Accreditation is done by the Joint Commission, AABB, and other state and federal agencies. CLIA 88 or the Clinical Laboratory Improvement Amendments also dictate testing and personnel.

The accrediting body in Australia is NATA, all laboratories must be NATA accredited to receive payment from Medicare.

New realities are placing pressures on the healthcare industry, and how patient care is delivered. Rising hospital management costs, an aging population, a shortage of healthcare workers, challenges in accessing services, timely availability of information, issues of safety and quality, and rising consumerism are some of the facts of today's healthcare system. The industry has reached a point of chasm, where they need to decide how services could be delivered more effectively to reduce costs, improve quality, and extend reach. The critical questions facing the industry today include: how can we effectively manage hospitals and provide enhanced services without placing additional burden on a system already pushed to its limits; how can we provide care in a cost-efficient manner at a time when healthcare spending is rising; and how do we most efficiently use our resources and support front-line staff in order to reduce medical errors and enhance quality of care.

These are just a few questions facing the industry. It looks bleak, but there's hope. There are new information technologies available to help. Information technologies that enable immediate, information-rich communications and provide easy-to-use collaborative tools are increasingly becoming a vital part of today's healthcare.

Laboratory medicine is the keystone on which the structure of scientific medicine is erected. A wide variety of laboratory-based disciplines (e.g., histology, hematology, clinical chemistry, Immunology and microbiology) contribute to nearly all of the elements necessary to effectively control infectious and noninfectious diseases. The clinical laboratory is no longer its own limited bionetwork, as it is increasingly integrated with patient care, assisting diagnosis, monitoring therapies and predicting clinical outcomes. A lack of reliable and efficient laboratory service can result in serious consequences for the patients as well as obscuring the true picture of the problem in an entire country.

Clinical laboratories have achieved significant improvements in the provision and quality of diagnostic tests. Automation, commercially produced reagents and computers are providing clinicians with an ever-increasing list of rapid and cost-effective tests. Advances in laboratory medicine have occurred in concert with analytical developments that measure many different molecules with specificity for pathological conditions, and with ever-increasing sensitivity. Such tests have revolutionized clinical diagnosis in ways that were unimaginable even a decade ago. As a consequence, laboratorians and their departments, at least in most developed countries, are expected to meet stringent technical, management and quality-assurance standards.

Laboratory Services in Developing Countries

It is unfortunate that the number and quality of clinical laboratories in developing countries leave a lot to be desired. Although a few top-of-the-line laboratories in these countries compare favorably with those in developed nations, their number is very small. However the vast majority of patients do not have routine access to such laboratories.

In many developing countries, opening a laboratory is as easy as opening a grocery store - or rather, opening a grocery store may be more complicated! A clinical laboratory can be established without requiring permission from any government or professional association. There is no paperwork since there are no regulations governing the management or quality of laboratory practice and in some countries, no license is needed. The factors determining the performance of a clinical laboratory include good equipment, reliable reagents and trained, conscientious staff, but many laboratories compromise on such vital prerequisites. In many cases, retired laboratory technicians and other, often entirely unqualified people, open small clinical laboratories, where standards are not maintained since their knowledge is limited. The managers earn money by using outdated machines, compromising on the reagents and by employing technicians in place of clinical pathologists able to interpret the test results properly and to ensure the achievement of minimal technical standards. Yet the medical laboratory should provide a vital part of the management of any patient – any lapse or mistake in the performance of tests can lead to serious harm whether at the diagnostic stage or in the course of treatment.

Causes of Poor Laboratory Services in Developing Countries

There are numerous causes of poor services, the primary one being failure to follow regulations, or in some cases, to develop relevant regulations. The reasons for this are many and varied but professional laboratory staff as a whole must share the responsibility for tolerating inefficient or obviously incorrect practices. The following factors are especially relevant:

Low Budget: In most developing countries including Egypt, health care is primarily funded from general government revenue without charging the consumers. The expenditure on health is very low to begin with. It is less than one quarter of what developed countries spend and often very much less. Moreover its distribution amongst the various sectors is inequitable. Most funding is spent on high-profile projects in teaching institutions in large urban centres. Laboratory services do not command a high priority.

Scarcity of Laboratory Staff: The tremendous progress in the field of laboratory medicine has made accurate assessment and monitoring the progress of an ailment much easier. The result has been a great rush in demand for laboratory services. It is unfortunate that the availability of laboratory personnel has lagged far behind. In addition, there is significant migration of trained manpower to more profitable markets abroad.

The exact number of clinical laboratory staff working in Egypt, their background and qualifications has not been determined. However, according to one estimate, there are no more than 1500 clinical pathologists, or about 10 per million of the Pakistan population. By contrast, a developed country, such as England, has 109 pathologists per million. Support staff, such as technicians, is in even shorter supply. In Afghanistan there are hardly any at all. In Brazil, until a few years ago, pathologists outnumbered technologists. There is no doubt that a huge gap exists between supply and demand.

Poor Training: The training of pathologists and technicians leaves much to be desired. Most general pathologists have received as little as nine months training in four major subjects. Only in recent years has training been improved to acceptable standards. Similarly, many technicians receive only on-the-job training, with little formal education. The quality of the work of such a body of inadequately trained personnel is bound to be substandard.

Lack of Appropriate Equipment and Infrastructure: Laboratory equipment is mostly manufactured in industrialized countries. It has become increasingly more sophisticated. The procurement officials in developing countries usually buy such fancy gadgetry for purposes of prestige rather than to make full use of its capabilities. There is no infrastructure for maintenance, or even an assured supply of electricity. It is therefore not surprising that developing countries are known as graveyards of equipment. It takes less than one year for some machines to break down in some way and approximately 60-80% of laboratory equipment is estimated to be non-functional.

Lack of Regulatory Mechanisms: There is no license required to establish a clinical laboratory in many developing countries. In Southeast Asian regions of the World Health Organization (WHO), only two out of seven countries had accreditation programs. There are no rules or training requirements for non-pathologist physicians who run or lend their names to laboratories.

Lack of Continuing Education: At present there is almost no provision for continuing education for pathologists. It is usually not required by the institutions that initially award them degrees. The result is that most do not keep up with advances in the field. Yet in such a fast-moving area, it is important that clinical pathologists remain up-to-date with ever-changing technology.

Steps Necessary for Improvement of* in vitro *Diagnostics in Developing Countries

A number of steps are required of governments as well as professional associations to improve to the current situation:

External Quality Assessment (EQA): A system of EQA including laboratory licensure, accreditation, certification and proficiency testing has to be introduced to provide recognition to those who conform to acceptable standards.

The current international requirements would perhaps be too stringent for the vast majority of existing labs. It may be necessary to evolve a system by which such laboratories are included in a simpler quality assurance program and are gradually brought up to international standards over a period of time.

Training larger numbers of qualified Laboratory Staff: As the number of qualified staff is small, their place is taken up by unqualified non-medicals/untrained physicians. The supply of qualified staff can be increased by providing more training opportunities both within the developing countries themselves and, in some cases, abroad (although this is more expensive and entails the risk of economic migration). It may be helpful to arrange short visits by foreign experts.

Telecommunication: In view of the inadequate supply of trained laboratory staff, telecommunication could provide immediate relief by making expertise available electronically via the Internet or multiple telephone lines in far flung areas. This approach could also be used at an international level for both consultations and training, including continuing education.

Suitable Technologies for Developing Countries: There is a plethora of in vitro diagnostic devices available in more developed countries. Equipment and reagents appropriate to the needs of developing countries should be introduced. A system similar to WHO's essential drug list (essential laboratory tests) has been proposed. Laboratory staff should be trained in such techniques that are less expensive and require less elaborate infra-structure and equipment such that they could be more rapidly and more widely introduced.

The improvement in laboratory services will be a slow process: It is however imperative that a beginning is made so that the suffering of patients is reduced and disease control is brought onto a more rational and firmer footing.

Organize National Structures to Support a Countrywide Laboratory Quality System

National structures capable of supporting a quality system for laboratories at country level will require the following measures:

The placement of skilled laboratory scientists/managers with sufficient authority in leadership positions in the ministries of health;

Creation of a national laboratory quality office and appointment of a quality officer with authority and responsibility for oversight of national laboratory quality programmes;

The allocation of adequate financial resources to ensure compliance with national quality programmes.

Establish National Laboratory Quality Standards

International efforts are under way to develop health laboratory standards that help to ensure quality. These efforts should be supported as follows:

Each country should establish its own set of standards according to country-specific needs based on internationally agreed standards.

National laboratory standards need to take into account local factors, including any pertinent regulations, organization of the country's laboratory system(s), and resource constraints.

It is recommended that countries with limited resources consider taking a staged approach, where principal requirements for all are stated in the national laboratory standards as a minimum requirement while more advanced and national reference laboratories are encouraged to aim at meeting internationally accepted standards such as ISO 15189.

Implement Major Laboratory Quality System Programmes

Many activities associated with quality assurance must be carried out by local laboratories, but assistance and oversight will be required at the national level. The following activities should be planned at a national level, with help and input from laboratories throughout the country, to:

- establish and revise national quality standards;
- ensure that laboratory facilities and infrastructure are adequate and properly maintained for all testing being performed;
- ensure safety in all health laboratory facilities to protect workers within the laboratory, visitors to the facility and the general public at large;
- establish long-range plans for ensuring adequate and sustainable numbers of properly trained personnel for conducting laboratory operations;
- apply appropriate quality systems to all parts of laboratory management and operations, including the procurement
- process for supplies and equipment;
- develop national resources for ensuring internal quality control and for external quality assessment;
- develop a process for monitoring laboratory performance improvement;
- encourage the development of a structured advisory network for laboratories.

Social and Legal Aspects of Health Care Management

The modern face of medicine reflects a prodigious and growing range of treatment options. Paralleling this growth, society is witnessing an expanding acceptance of respect for patient autonomy in healthcare decision-making. While acknowledging that active patient involvement in medical management can lead to a more successful outcome, physicians can become frustrated when their advice is ignored or rejected by patients. This dynamic has created both a partnership and tension in the doctor-patient relationship. In England and Scotland, a body of law has developed which has begun to sort out the complex issues that can arise when patients, families and physicians disagree.

Medico- Legal Aspects of the Usage of Electronic Health Record

In the recent years, healthcare organizations are showing an increased rate of acquisition of computer technologies and their spending rates shows an upward tendency placing the industry as one to the major consumers of ICT products and services. Frost & Sullivan estimates the Health Information Technology market (by revenue) in 2008, in APAC (Southeast Asia, China, Japan and Australia) was close to USD5.04 billion with an annual growth rate (CAGR) of 11.8 percent from 2005-2008. Although the APAC HIT market represents currently only 2.1 percent of the total healthcare market, it is very likely that the figure could double if not triple that in the next 10 years.

Dr. Pawel Suwinsk, senior consultant at Frost & Sullivan says, 'The HIT is here to stay with even more ubiquitous presence in all aspects of healthcare delivery systems. Moreover, it will be the main factor and driver in the transformation of healthcare industry towards translation care by providing common collaboration platform for information processing and exchange between related sciences and industries.'

He further elaborates, " 50 percent of the medical practice activities can be controlled. The remaining 50 percent depends solely on human judgment and cognitive functions that when unfavourable conditions are present could lead to substandard care. The implementation of HIT can improve the quality of care by providing better control (up to 80 percent). However, while decreasing the legal exposure of traditional medical practice it introduces legal implications related to the usage of HIT." The following are some of the medico-legal aspects of the usage of healthcare IT solutions including electronic medical records.

Medical liability which is also entitled as medical negligence or medical malpractice is a special component of tort law which governs the professional relationship between physicians and their patients. It is concerned about the duties of care expected between physicians and their patients in delivering health care. It is said that the duty of a physician to his or her patients is to practice medicine which meets or exceeds the standard of care.

If the hospital or healthcare delivery organizations violate standard of care (through inadequate oversight of its staff physicians) by allowing EHR or other technology of its choice to be used in such a way to harm patients, it might become the subject of corporate negligence action. The case of Vicarious liability occurs when there is a design or other type of flaw in any of the technologies including electronic health record or computerized physician order entry that causes harm to patients even though the physicians or other caregivers who uses that committed no negligence.

The unauthorized access to patient's private information results in the privacy violation. User negligence, misdirected information flow or intentional security breach by a third party etc..could be some of the reasons for this information leakage. Security breached is recognized as unauthorized sharing of patient's private information. Inappropriate disclosure can happen in clinical setting when multiple copies of Electronic Health Record (EHR) persist even after destruction of original file is being accessed by unauthorized personnel.

Medical liability actions may also arise from acts of commission which breach the standard of care and result in injury and damages to patients. Physicians could also find themselves in trouble by failing to use diagnostic and treatment modalities suggested by the embedded best practice guidelines in certain types of electronic health records. Here there could be an act of omission contributing to patient injury.

Some of the preventative measures suggested in the course of medical liability are the selection of appropriate healthcare information system, proper training of staff to ensure efficient use of system, documenting all information with justification (whether or not care provided), and preventing any further alteration to this records without proper documentation etc..

Medical Ethics

Medical ethics is primarily a field of applied ethics, the study of moral values and judgments as they apply to medicine. As a scholarly discipline, medical ethics encompasses its practical application in clinical settings as well as work on its history, philosophy, theology, and sociology.

Medical ethics tends to be understood narrowly as an applied professional ethics, whereas bioethics appears to have worked more expansive concerns, touching upon the philosophy of science and issues of biotechnology. Still, the two fields often overlap and the distinction is more a matter of style than professional consensus. Medical ethics shares many principles with other branches of healthcare ethics, such as nursing ethics.

History

Historically, Western medical ethics may be traced to guidelines on the duty of physicians in antiquity, such as the Hippocratic Oath, and early rabbinic and Christian teachings. In the medieval and early modern period, the field is indebted to Muslim physicians such as Ishaq bin Ali Rahawi (who wrote the *Conduct of a Physician*, the first book dedicated to medical ethics) and Muhammad ibn Zakariya ar-Razi (known as Rhazes in the West), Jewish thinkers such as Maimonides, Roman Catholic scholastic thinkers such as Thomas Aquinas, and the case-oriented analysis (casuistry) of Catholic moral theology. These intellectual traditions continue in Catholic, Islamic and Jewish medical ethics.

By the 18th and 19th centuries, medical ethics emerged as a more self-conscious discourse. For instance, authors such as Thomas Percival wrote about "medical jurisprudence" and reportedly coined the phrase "medical ethics." Percival's guidelines related to physician consultations have been criticized as being excessively protective of the home physician's reputation. Jeffrey Berlant is one such critic who considers Percival's codes of physician consultations as being an early example of the anti-competitive, "guild"-like nature of the physician community. In 1847, the American Medical Association adopted its first code of ethics, with this being based in large part upon Percival's work. While the secularized field borrowed largely from Catholic medical ethics, in the 20th century a distinctively liberal Protestant approach was articulated by thinkers such as Joseph Fletcher. In the 1960s and 1970s, building upon liberal theory and procedural justice, much of the discourse of medical ethics went through a dramatic shift and largely reconfigured itself into bioethics.

Since the 1970s, the growing influence of ethics in contemporary medicine can be seen in the increasing use of Institutional Review Boards to evaluate experiments on human subjects, the establishment of hospital ethics committees, the expansion of the role of clinician ethicists, and the integration of ethics into many medical school curricula.

Values in Medical Ethics

Six of the values that commonly apply to medical ethics discussions are:

- Autonomy - the patient has the right to refuse or choose their treatment.
- Beneficence - a practitioner should act in the best interest of the patient.
- Non-maleficence - "first, do no harm".
- Justice - concerns the distribution of scarce health resources, and the decision of who gets what treatment (fairness and equality).
- Dignity - the patient (and the person treating the patient) have the right to dignity.
- Truthfulness and honesty - the concept of informed consent has increased in importance since the historical events of the Doctors' Trial of the Nuremberg trials and Tuskegee Syphilis Study.

Values such as these do not give answers as to how to handle a particular situation, but provide a useful framework for understanding conflicts.

When moral values are in conflict, the result may be an ethical dilemma or crisis. Sometimes, no good solution to a dilemma in medical ethics exists, and occasionally, the values of the medical community (i.e., the hospital and its staff) conflict with the values of the individual patient, family, or larger non-medical community.

Conflicts can also arise between health care providers, or among family members. Some argue for example, that the principles of autonomy and beneficence clash when patients refuse blood transfusions, considering them life-saving; and truth-telling was not emphasized to a large extent before the HIV era.

Autonomy

The principle of autonomy recognizes the rights of individuals to self determination. This is rooted in society's respect for individuals' ability to make informed decisions about personal matters. Autonomy has become more important as social values have shifted to define medical quality in terms of outcomes that are important to the patient rather than medical professionals. The increasing importance of autonomy can be seen as a social reaction to a "paternalistic" tradition within healthcare. Some have questioned whether the backlash against historically excessive paternalism in favour of patient autonomy has inhibited the proper use of soft paternalism to the detriment of outcomes for some patients. Respect for autonomy is the basis for informed consent and advance directives.

Autonomy is a general indicator of health. Many diseases are characterised by loss of autonomy, in various manners. This makes autonomy an indicator for both personal well-being, and for the well-being of the profession. This has implications for the consideration of medical ethics: "is the aim of health care to do good, and benefit from it?"; or "is the aim of health care to do good to others, and have them, and society, benefit from this?". (Ethics - by definition - tries to find a beneficial balance between the activities of the individual and its effects on a collective.)

By considering Autonomy as a gauge parameter for (self) health care, the medical and ethical perspective both benefit from the implied reference to Health.

Beneficence

The term beneficence refers to actions that promote the wellbeing of others. In the medical context, this means taking actions that serve the best interests of patients. However, uncertainty surrounds the precise definition of which practices do in fact help patients.

James Childress and Tom Beauchamp in *Principle of Biomedical Ethics* (1978) identify beneficence as one of the core values of health care ethics. Some scholars, such as Edmund Pellegrino, argue that beneficence is the *only* fundamental principle of medical ethics. They argue that healing should be the sole purpose of medicine, and that endeavors like cosmetic surgery, contraception and euthanasia fall beyond its purview.

Non-Maleficence

The concept of non-maleficence is embodied by the phrase, "first, do no harm," or the Latin, *primum non nocere*. Many consider that should be the main or primary consideration (hence *primum*): that it is more important not to harm your patient, than to do them good. This is partly because enthusiastic practitioners are prone to using treatments that they believe will do good, without first having evaluated them adequately to ensure they do no (or only acceptable levels of) harm. Much harm has been done to patients as a result. It is not only more important to do no harm than to do good; it is also important to *know* how likely it is that your treatment will harm a patient. So a physician should go further than not prescribing medications they know to be harmful - he or she should not prescribe medications (or otherwise treat the patient) unless s/he knows that the treatment is unlikely to be harmful; or at the very least, that patient understands the risks and benefits, and that the likely benefits outweigh the likely risks.

In practice, however, many treatments carry some risk of harm. In some circumstances, e.g. in desperate situations where the outcome without treatment will be grave, risky treatments that stand a high chance of harming the patient will be justified, as the risk of not treating is also very likely to do harm. So the principle of *non-maleficence* is not absolute, and must be balanced against the principle of *beneficence* (doing good).

"Non-maleficence" is defined by its cultural context. Every culture has its own cultural collective definitions of 'good' and 'evil'. Their definitions depend on the degree to which the culture sets its cultural values apart from nature. In some cultures the terms "good" and "evil" are absent: for them these words lack meaning as their experience of nature does not set them apart from nature. Other cultures place the humans in interaction with nature, some even place humans in a position of dominance over nature. The religions are the main means of expression of these considerations.

Depending on the cultural consensus conditioning (expressed by its religious, political and legal social system) the legal definition of Non-maleficence differs. Violation of non-maleficence is the subject of medical malpractice litigation. Regulations thereof differ, over time, per nation.

Double Effect

Some interventions undertaken by physicians can create a positive outcome while foreseeably, but unintentionally, doing harm. The combination of these two circumstances is known as the "double effect". A commonly cited, but fallacious, example of this phenomenon is the use of morphine in the dying patient. Such use of morphine can ease the pain and suffering of the patient, while simultaneously hastening the demise of the patient through suppression of the respiratory drive. If correct, this would be an example of the double effect; however, no research evidence supports the claim that appropriately administered opioid drugs depress the respiratory system.

Conflicts between Autonomy and Beneficence/Non-maleficence

Autonomy can come into conflict with Beneficence when patients disagree with recommendations that health care professionals believe are in the patient's best interest. When the patient's interests conflict with the patient's welfare, different societies settle the conflict in a wide range of manners. Western medicine generally defers to the wishes of a mentally competent patient to make his own decisions, even in cases where the medical team believes that he is not acting in his own best interests. However, many other societies prioritize beneficence over autonomy.

Examples include when a patient does not want a treatment because of, for example, religious or cultural views. In the case of euthanasia, the patient, or relatives of a patient, may want to end the life of the patient. Also, the patient may want an unnecessary treatment, as can be the case in hypochondria. A doctor may want to prefer Autonomy because refusal to please the patient's will would harm the doctor-patient relationship. Individuals' capacity for informed decision making may come into question during resolution of conflicts between Autonomy and Beneficence. The role of surrogate medical decision makers is an extension of the principle of autonomy.

Euthanasia

Some American physicians interpret the non-maleficence principle to exclude the practice of euthanasia, though not all concur. Probably the most extreme example in recent history of the violation of the non-maleficence dictum was Dr. Jack Kevorkian, who was convicted of second-degree homicide in Michigan in 1998 after demonstrating active euthanasia on the TV news show, 60 Minutes.

In some countries euthanasia is accepted as standard medical practice. Legal regulations assign this to the medical profession. In such nations, the aim is to alleviate the suffering of patients from diseases known to be incurable by the methods known in that culture. In that sense, the "Primum no Nocere" is based on the realisation that *the inability of the medical expert to offer help, creates a known great and ongoing suffering in the patient*. "Not acting" in those cases is believed to be more damaging than actively relieving the suffering of the patient. Evidently the ability to offer help depends on the limitation of what the practitioner can do. These limitations are characteristic for each different form of healing, and the legal system of the specific culture. The aim to "not do harm" is still the same. It gives the medical practitioner a responsibility to help the patient, in the intentional and active relief of suffering, in those cases where no cure can be offered.

Informed Consent

Informed consent in ethics usually refers to the idea that a person must be fully-informed about and understand the potential benefits and risks of their choice of treatment. An uninformed person is at risk of mistakenly making a choice not reflective of his or her values or wishes. It does not specifically mean the process of obtaining consent, nor the specific legal requirements, which vary from place to place, for capacity to consent. Patients can elect to make their own medical decisions, or can delegate decision-making authority to another party. If the patient is incapacitated, laws around the world designate different processes for obtaining informed consent, typically by having a person appointed by the patient or their next of kin make decisions for them. The value of informed consent is closely related to the values of autonomy and truth telling.

A correlate to "informed consent" is the concept of informed refusal.

Confidentiality

Confidentiality is commonly applied to conversations between doctors and patients. This concept is commonly known as patient-physician privilege.

Legal protections prevent physicians from revealing their discussions with patients, even under oath in court.

Confidentiality is mandated in America by HIPAA laws, specifically the Privacy Rule, and various state laws, some more rigorous than HIPAA. However, numerous exceptions to the rules have been carved out over the years. For example, many states require physicians to report gunshot wounds to the police and impaired drivers to the Department of Motor Vehicles. Confidentiality is also challenged in cases involving the diagnosis of a sexually transmitted disease in a patient who refuses to reveal the diagnosis to a spouse, and in the termination of a pregnancy in an underage patient, without the knowledge of the patient's parents. Many states in the U.S. have laws governing parental notification in underage abortion.

Traditionally, medical ethics has viewed the duty of confidentiality as a relatively non-negotiable tenet of medical practice. More recently, critics like Jacob Appel have argued for a more nuanced approach to the duty that acknowledges the need for flexibility in many cases.

Criticisms of Orthodox Medical Ethics

It has been argued that mainstream medical ethics is biased by the assumption of a framework in which individuals are not simply free to contract with one another to provide whatever medical treatment is demanded, subject to the ability to pay. Because a high proportion of medical care is typically provided via the welfare state, and because there are legal restrictions on what treatment may be provided and by whom, an automatic divergence may exist between the wishes of patients and the preferences of medical practitioners and other parties. Tassano has questioned the idea that Beneficence might in some cases have priority over Autonomy. He argues that violations of Autonomy more often reflect the interests of the state or of the supplier group than those of the patient.

Routine regulatory professional bodies or the courts of law are valid social recourses.

Importance of Communication

Many so-called "ethical conflicts" in medical ethics are traceable back to a lack of communication. Communication breakdowns between patients and their healthcare team, between family members, or between members of the medical community, can all lead to disagreements and strong feelings. These breakdowns should be remedied, and many apparently insurmountable "ethics" problems can be solved with open lines of communication.

Control and Resolution

To ensure that appropriate ethical values are being applied within hospitals, effective hospital accreditation requires that ethical considerations are taken into account, for example with respect to physician integrity, conflicts of interest, research ethics and organ transplantation ethics.

Guidelines

There are various ethical guidelines. For example, the Declaration of Helsinki is regarded as authoritative in human research ethics.

In the United Kingdom, General Medical Council provides clear overall modern guidance in the form of its 'Good Medical Practice' statement. Other organisations, such as the Medical Protection Society and a number of university departments, are often consulted by British doctors regarding issues relating to ethics.

Ethics Committees

Often, simple communication is not enough to resolve a conflict, and a hospital ethics committee must convene to decide a complex matter. These bodies are composed primarily of health care professionals, but may also include philosophers, lay people, and clergy - indeed, in many parts of the world their presence is considered mandatory in order to provide balance.

With respect to the expected composition of such bodies in the USA, Europe and Australia, the following applies.

U.S. recommendations suggest that Research and Ethical Boards (REBs) should have five or more members, including at least one scientist, one non-scientist and one person not affiliated with the institution. The REB should include people knowledgeable in the law and standards of practice and professional conduct. Special memberships are advocated for handicapped or disabled concerns, if required by the protocol under review.

The European Forum for Good Clinical Practice (EFGCP) suggests that REBs include two practicing physicians who share experience in biomedical research and are independent from the institution where the research is conducted; one lay person; one lawyer; and one paramedical professional, e.g. nurse or pharmacist. They recommend that a quorum include both sexes from a wide age range and reflect the cultural make-up of the local community.

The 1996 Australian Health Ethics Committee recommendations were entitled, "Membership Generally of Institutional Ethics Committees". They suggest a chairperson be preferably someone not employed or otherwise connected with the institution. Members should include a person with knowledge and experience in professional care, counselling or treatment of humans; a minister of religion or equivalent, e.g. Aboriginal elder; a layman; a laywoman; a lawyer and, in the case of a hospital-based ethics committee, a nurse.

The assignment of philosophers or religious clerics will reflect the importance attached by the society to the basic values involved. An example from Sweden with Torbjorn Tannsjo on a couple of such committees indicates secular trends gaining influence.

Cultural Concerns

Culture differences can create difficult medical ethics problems. Some cultures have spiritual or magical theories about the origins of disease, for example, and reconciling these beliefs with the tenets of Western medicine can be difficult.

Truth-telling

Some cultures do not place a great emphasis on informing the patient of the diagnosis, especially when cancer is the diagnosis. Even American culture did not emphasize truth-telling in a cancer case, up until the 1970s. In American medicine, the principle of informed consent takes precedence over other ethical values, and patients are usually at least asked whether they want to know the diagnosis.

Online Business Practices

The delivery of diagnosis online leads patients to believe that doctors in some parts of the country are at the direct service of drug companies. Finding diagnosis as convenient as what drug still has patent rights on it. Physicians and drug companies are found to be competing for top ten search engine ranks to lower costs of selling these drugs with little to no patient involvement.

Conflicts of Interest

Physicians should not allow a conflict of interest to influence medical judgment. In some cases, conflicts are hard to avoid, and doctors have a responsibility to avoid entering such situations. Unfortunately, research has shown that conflicts of interests are very common among both academic physicians and physicians in practice. The Pew Charitable Trusts has announced the Prescription Project for "academic medical centres, professional medical societies and public and private payers to end conflicts of interest resulting from the $12 billion spent annually on pharmaceutical marketing".

Referral

For example, doctors who receive income from referring patients for medical tests have been shown to refer more patients for medical tests. This practice is proscribed by the American

College of Physicians Ethics Manual. Fee splitting and the payments of commissions to attract referrals of patients is considered unethical and unacceptable in most parts of the world - while it is rapidly becoming routine in other countries, like India, where many urban practitioners currently pay a percentage of office-visit charges, lab tests as well as hospital care to unaccredited "quacks", or semi-accredited "practitioners of alternative medicine", who refer the patient. It is tolerated in some areas of US medical care as well.

Vendor Relationships

Studies show that doctors can be influenced by drug company inducements, including gifts and food. Industry-sponsored Continuing Medical Education (CME) programs influence prescribing patterns. Many patients surveyed in one study agreed that physician gifts from drug companies influence prescribing practices. A growing movement among physicians is attempting to diminish the influence of pharmaceutical industry marketing upon medical practice, as evidenced by Stanford University's ban on drug company-sponsored lunches and gifts. Other academic institutions that have banned pharmaceutical industry-sponsored gifts and food include the University of Pennsylvania, and Yale University.

Treatment of Family Members

Many doctors treat their family members. Doctors who do so must be vigilant not to create conflicts of interest or treat inappropriately.

Sexual Relationships

Sexual relationships between doctors and patients can create ethical conflicts, since sexual consent may conflict with the fiduciary responsibility of the physician. Doctors who enter into sexual relationships with patients face the threats of deregistration and prosecution.

In the early 1990s it was estimated that 2-9% of doctors had violated this rule Sexual relationships between physicians and patients' relatives may also be prohibited in some jurisdictions, although this prohibition is highly controversial.

Futility

The concept of medical futility has been an important topic in discussions of medical ethics. What should be done if there is no chance that a patient will survive but the family members insist on advanced care? Previously, some articles defined futility as the patient having less than a one percent chance of surviving. Some of these cases wind up in the courts. Advanced directives include living wills and durable powers of attorney for health care. In many cases, the "expressed wishes" of the patient are documented in these directives, and this provides a framework to guide family members and health care professionals in the decision making process when the patient is incapacitated. Undocumented expressed wishes can also help guide decisions in the absence of advanced directives, as in the Quinlan case in Missouri.

"Substituted judgment" is the concept that a family member can give consent for treatment if the patient is unable (or unwilling) to give consent himself. The key question for the decision making surrogate is not, "What would you like to do?", but instead, "What do you think the patient would want in this situation?".

Courts have supported family's arbitrary definitions of futility to include simple biological survival, as in the Baby K case (in which the courts ordered a child born with only a brain stem instead of a complete brain to be kept on a ventilator based on the religious belief that all life must be preserved).

In some hospitals, medical futility is referred to as "non-beneficial care."

Baby Doe Law establishes state protection for a disabled child's right to life, ensuring that this right is protected even over the wishes of parents or guardians in cases where they want to withhold treatment.

Quality of Life (Healthcare)

Quality of life (QOL) is used in healthcare to refer to an individual's emotional, social and physical wellbeing, including their ability to function in the ordinary tasks of living. It is a term used most frequently in the context of medicine and healthcare, where the impact of a disease may reduce "Health-related Quality of Life"

Understanding quality of life is recognized as increasingly important in healthcare,, where the relationship between cost and value raises complex problems. For instance, health providers must make economic decisions about access to expensive drugs that may prolong life by a few months, and weight these against alternative uses such as preventative medicine or a surgical bed. Monetary measures alone do not readily apply. In the case of chronic and/or terminal illness where there is no effective treatment or cure, there may be an emphasis on improving HRQoL through interventions such as symptom management, adaptive technology, and palliative care. There is a growing field of research concerned with developing, evaluating and applying quality of life measures within health related research (e.g. within randomized controlled trials), especially Health Services Research. Well-executed HRQoL research informs those tasked with health rationing, is involved in the decision-making process of bodies such as the Food and Drug Administration or National Institute for Clinical Excellence, and may be used as an endpoint in clinical trials of experimental therapies.

Initial QoL measures referred to simple assessments of physical abilities by an external rater (e.g.: patient is able to get up, eat and drink, take care of personal hygiene without any help by others), or even to a single measurement (e.g. the angle to which a limb could be flexed).

The current concept of HRQoL acknowledges that subjects put their actual situation in relation to their individual expectation. The latter can vary over time, and react to external influences like long-time disease, family support etc. Patients' and e.g. physicians' rating of the same objective situation have been found to differ significantly. Consequently, HRQoL is nowadays usually assessed using patient questionnaires. These are often multidimensional and cover physical, social, emotional, cognitive, work- or role-related, and possibly spiritual aspects as well as a wide variety of disease related symptoms, therapy induced side-effects, and even the financial impact of medical conditions.

Hundreds of validated QoL questionnaires have been developed: Generic instruments (e.g. SF-36, Short-Form with 36 questions) as well as disease specific instruments (e.g. the LC-13 Lung Cancer module from the EORTC Quality of Life questionnaire library, or the HADS Hospital Anxiety and Depression Scale). Like other psychometric assessment tools, QoL questionnaires should meet certain quality criteria, most importantly with regard to their reliability and validity.

"Improved Quality of Life" is also often advertised for marketing purposes. This is not limited to the medical field; but here, the growing impact of chronic conditions that cannot ultimately be healed, but merely controlled or made bearable, adds to the relevance of the topic.

Frequently Used HRQoL Measures

- Short-Form Health Survey One example of a widely-used questionnaire assessing physical, social, and mental HRQoL, used in clinical trials.
- Manchester Short Assessment of Quality of Life 16-item questionnaire for use in psychiatric populations.
- EQ-5D a simple quality of life questionnaire.

The quality of life ethic refers to an ethical principle which uses assessments of the quality of life that a person can experience or hope to experience as a foundation for making decisions about the continuation or termination of life. It is often used in contrast to or in opposition to the sanctity of life ethic.

5

Nursing Administration and Management

Traditionally, the purpose of nursing administration has been to design, manage, and facilitate patient care delivery. Nurse managers assume leadership roles in planning, organizing, and implementing care for people across the broad spectrum of health care settings. The aspects of quality outcomes, staff development, care management, strategic planning, and research are within the conceptual framework of nursing management and leadership.

Administrative nursing personnel may include three types of managers:

1. first-line managers who are directly responsible for producing nursing services; they are typically known as nurse managers or primary care nurses
2. middle managers who coordinate the work of several units; job titles are coordinators, clinical nurse managers, or case managers
3. nurse executives who are responsible for the overall operations of patient care services; titles are directors of patient care services or executive vice presidents for nursing.

The setting for nurse managers has been changing as a result of prospective payment, reduced admissions, and reduced length of stay. With the expansion of nursing care into outpatient clinics, surgi-centres, and home health care, nursing administrators in these areas are taking on additional responsibilities for contract negotiation, corporate access for support services, and management of interdisciplinary services.

Education for nurse administrators can be acquired in a variety of ways: preparation at the degree level—master's of science in nursing or master's of health administration, business administration, or public administration; certificate programs that may or may not require a master's prerequisite; or informal programs such as facility-sponsored management programs, self-study, continuing education, or national certification exams.

The science of nursing administration has its roots with Florence Nightingale's systematic organization for patient care. Historically, nursing administration is grounded in the study by Herman Finer seeking ways to improve nursing services in hospitals. Findings from this study led to further demonstration projects that identified the theories, concepts, and principles of nursing administration, as well as established the graduate curricula for the discipline.

Nursing administration is considered to be an applied science and includes components of clinical nursing care, collaborative practice, and management theories and concepts. Today, as nurse administrators respond to changes in health care systems from market forces, political pressures, and consumer demands, nursing administration practice is a compilation of various management practices and theories.

Discussion

This study found that nursing administration authors cite the core titles in nursing administration most often, as four of the five analyzed journals were found to be the top four journal titles cited in Zone 1. *Seminars for Nurse Managers,* the newest nursing administration title, was found in Zone 2, not surprising because it began publication in 1993 and the time frame for publication was 1996 to 1998. As a newcomer to the nursing administration literature, it did not have a strong showing based on citation analysis. The remaining five journals in Zone 1—*American Journal of Nursing, Nursing Research, Hospitals & Health Networks, New*

England Journal of Medicine, and *JAMA*—reflected the research, administrative, and clinical management functions of nursing managers and administrators.

Nursing administration literature deals with many "hot topics" as well as legal, ethical, and clinical issues, and this was reflected in the number of references to weekly journals—*Hospital & Health Networks, JAMA,* and *New England Journal of Medicine.* The broad scope of nursing administration could be seen in Zone 2, where sixty-six titles reflected these subject categories: clinical nursing, administrative nursing, nursing research, health care administration, general business, social sciences, psychology, and medicine.

Conclusion

Searching the core databases of PubMed/Medlineand Cinahl will provide fairly comprehensive coverage of this discipline. Nurse administrators and managers need to search PubMed/ MEDLINE to supplement CINAHL's limited indexing coverage of medical titles—such as *JAMA, New England Journal of Medicine,* and the *Annals of Internal Medicine*—and certain core health care management titles—particularly *Hospitals & Health Networks, Modern Healthcare,* and *Medical Care.* Trends in leadership and management theory are borrowed heavily from the business literature. It is important that nursing administration leaders use a business or social sciences literature index to identify articles in titles such as *Harvard Business Review, Fortune, Administrative Science Quarterly,* and *Academic Management Journal* for research on management and leadership topics, increasingly important to today's nursing administrator.

Management of Health and Hospitals Services

Healthcare is changing more rapidly than almost any other field. The field is changing in terms of how and where care is delivered, who is providing those services, and how that care is financed. Healthcare management requires talented people to manage the changes taking place. In their roles, healthcare executives have an opportunity to make a significant contribution to improving the health of the communities their organizations serve. With growing diversity in the healthcare system, executives are needed in many settings, including:

- Clinics
- Consulting firms
- Health insurance organizations
- Healthcare associations
- Hospitals
- Nursing homes
- Physician practices
- Mental health organizations
- Public health departments
- Rehabilitation centres
- Skilled nursing facilities
- Universities and research institutions.

Today, an estimated 100,000 people occupy health management positions at numerous organizational levels, from department head to chief executive officer. Requirements for senior-level positions in healthcare organizations are demanding, but these jobs also offer opportunities to improve the system of care giving.

If you choose a career in healthcare management, your first job might be an entry- to mid-level management position in a specialized area, such as:

- Finance
- Government relations
- Human resources
- Information systems
- Marketing and public affairs
- Material management (purchasing of equipment and supplies)
- Medical staff relations
- Patient care services
- Planning and development.

Growth and Salaries

Healthcare management is a huge, complex, and ever-changing field. In fact, healthcare services will increase 30 percent from 1996-2006 and will account for 3.1 million new jobs, the largest increase of any industry.

Hospital Executive Salary Information

Two-thirds of ACHE affiliates are employed in hospitals or hospital systems. Fifty-two percent hold positions at the chief executive, executive vice president, or vice president level. The data here correspond to the salary information requests our affiliates frequently address to the ACHE Healthcare Executive Career Resource Centre.

Healthcare Administration in the Military and Department of Veterans Affairs

There are many rewarding and exciting healthcare management careers offered through the uniformed services as well as the Department of Veterans Affairs. Click on the links for additional information.

- Army
- Navy
- Air Force
- Department of Veterans Affairs.

According to a major World Bank study of public hospitals (Barnum and Kutzin, 1993), the share of public sector health resources in developing countries consumed by hospitals ranges from 50 to 80 percent.

This manual seeks to help managers make the best use of these resources. By better understanding the costs of various activities, managers can improve the efficiency of various hospital departments, as well as hospital systems as a whole. Finally, the data can help national policy makers decide which curative care is best delivered in hospitals, and to examine the tradeoffs among various preventive, primary curative, and secondary curative services.

Cost Finding and Analysis as Management Tools

In both developing and industrialized countries, hospitals are viewed as vital and necessary community resources that should be managed for the benefit of the community . As such, hospital management has a responsibility to the community—to provide health care services that the community needs, at an acceptable level of quality, and at the least possible cost. Cost finding and analysis can help departmental managers, hospital administrators, and policymakers to determine how well their institutions meet these public needs.

Cost finding and cost analysis are the technique of allocating direct and indirect costs as explained in this manual. They are also the process of manipulating or rearranging the data or information in existing accounts in order to obtain the costs of services rendered by the hospital. As financial management techniques, cost finding and analysis help to furnish the necessary data for making more informed decisions concerning operations and infrastructure investments. If structured accurately, cost data can provide information on operational performance by cost centre. This information can be compared to budgeted performance expectations in order to identify problem areas that require immediate attention. These data give management the material to evaluate and modify operations if necessary. Moreover, knowledge of costs (both unit and total) can assists in planning for future budgets (as an indicator of efficiency) and to establish a schedule of charges for patient services. A hospital cannot set rates and charges which are realistically related to costs unless the cost finding system accurately allocates both direct and indirect costs to the appropriate cost centre. Finally, cost finding and analysis are also of value to management in ensuring that costs do not exceed available revenues and subsidies. It is the best available technique for accomplishing this.

Computation of Unit Costs Using Line-item Expenditure Data

Two fundamental items of financial data needed by a hospital manager are allocated costs by cost centre (a program or department within a hospital) and the unit cost of hospital services. A unit of hospital services may be as small as one meal, or as broad as an entire inpatient stay.

To perform these calculations precisely, the hospital needs an accurate and comprehensive financial accounting system.

In many hospitals, however, existing accounting systems have gaps, such as excluding some costs or lacking the data to relate the costs to specific cost centres. In these cases, estimates are needed.. It is organized based on seven steps for computing unit costs, a framework built on the procedures of the UNICEF manual for analysis of district health service costs and financing (Hanson and Gilson, 1996). The steps are:

1. Define the final product.
2. Define cost centres.
3. Identify the full cost for each input.
4. Assign inputs to cost centres.
5. Allocate all costs to final cost centres.
6. Compute total and unit cost for each final cost centre.
7. Report results.

In leading the reader through this framework, we explain what data elements are needed, how different cost items can be treated, and how costs can be computed in certain situations or cases. In each case, we discuss a set of problems that have been identified in various studies of specific countries. In addition, we work through examples of certain highlighted points.

What are the services or departments for which you are interested in computing unit costs?

Define Cost Centres

The next step for computing unit costs is to determine the centres of activity in the hospital to which direct and/or indirect costs will be assigned. The major direct cost categories of most departments include salaries, supplies, and other (purchased services such as dues, travel, and rents).

Indirect cost categories include depreciation and allocated costs of other departments.

The rationale for choosing centres of activity that correspond with the hospital's organizational and/or accounting structure is managerial. Hospitals are organized into departments and, since we want to strengthen the management of these departments, it is useful to have cost centres that correspond to the existing organizational structure of the hospital. This provides: (1) the road map by which costs can be routed, through the process of cost finding, to final cost centres; and (2) a framework for costing the distinct functions of each centre. Following this road map shows individual managers how they are using available resources in relation to what has been budgeted and the services that they are providing.

From an administrative standpoint, cost centres can be distinguished based on the nature of their work—patient care, intermediate clinical care and overhead centres. As explained below, some costs centres represent patient-centered activities (i.e., final or intermediate cost centres), while others are primarily for general services (i.e., overhead cost centres) such as housekeeping, laundry, maintenance, and the many other tasks necessary for the satisfactory operation of a complex organization like a hospital.

Patient Care: These cost centres are responsible for direct patient services, for example, wards or inpatient care units as a whole, or the ambulatory care centre.

Intermediate: These cost centres provide ancillary services to support inpatient units but are organized as separate departments. Examples include laboratory, pharmacy, and radiology.

Overhead: These cost centres provide overhead support services to both patient care and intermediate cost centres. Examples of departments are finance (accounts receivable, accounts payable, payroll, etc.), dietetics, and security.

Within each of the above groups, there are also decisions about how many cost centres to define. For example, if you are planning to analyze unit costs by ward, then you would need to treat each ward as a separate cost centre. Or, if you want to distinguish ancillary costs by (type (e.g., x-ray vs. clinical laboratory), then establish separate cost centres for each.

The aim of unit cost analysis is to allocate hospital costs (direct and indirect) to centres whose costs are to be measured. Typically, you will be computing the unit cost mainly for patient care centres (e.g. maternity wards, outpatient clinics, or pediatric units). However, in some instances, you may need to know the cost per lab test or drug prescription, in which case unit costs are computed for intermediate departments such as laboratory and pharmacy. On occasion, you may even need to know the unit cost of an overhead service, like dietetics, if, for example, you are considering opening a competitive bidding process to contract food services rather than keeping it in-house, or you wish to compare the performance of dietetic departments across different hospitals.

In order to see the extent to which user charges (e.g., fees for room, board, and nursing [a daily rate inclusive of diagnostic and therapeutic services], drugs and dressings, x-ray laboratory, and physical therapy) cover their associated costs, it may be necessary to have a cost analysis system that identifies cost centres which produce revenue (i.e., patient care and intermediate cost centres) and general cost centres that do not produce revenue (e.g. security, housekeeping and payroll). This identification is necessary when it is desirable to allocate all direct or indirect expenses incurred by the general cost centre (non-revenue-producing centres) to revenue-producing centres which could be the final cost centres.

Finally, one may eventually want to compute two types of unit costs: with or without allocated ancillary amounts. For example, if calculating the cost per admission or inpatient stay, one figure could include laboratory and x-ray costs and one excluding them.

Identify the Full Cost for Each Input

An important part of computing unit costs is to make sure that you have cost data which are as complete as possible. Two issues are involved: (1) the conceptual issue of determining which expenditures should be counted as costs based on an economic sense of resources used up during production of health care, and

(2) the actual measurement of true costs using available data (which may be incomplete or untrustworthy). Various studies have developed ways to impute or approximate cost when existing data are problematic, and we describe some of these. Since the problems and responses often differ according to the line item, our discussion is partly organized by line item (e.g. drugs and salaries).

Salaries: To calculate the full or total cost of salaries, one should ideally use actual salary amounts paid to hospital employees. Sometimes these data may not be available such as in cases where employees are paid by the Ministry of Health and therefore the hospital cannot access this payroll data.

However, as some studies have shown, individual salaries can be approximated by using the midpoint of the salary range of the employee's classification level. In the Mills' study on hospitals in Malawi, the midpoint estimation approach appeared reasonable given that the estimated total wage costs was similar to the hospital's true wage costs. On the other hand, another study has shown that using the midpoint estimation approach may not accurately reflect true salaries. Researchers in Nigeria obtained data on the mean salary for each job classification across all hospitals and found it was consistently lower than the midpoint often by as much as 30%. Reanalyzing their data, we determined that using the midpoint in this study would have overstated true payroll cost by around 35%.

In some hospitals, salary information on certain expatriate staff may be hard to obtain since they are paid by foreign donor agencies with salaries denominated in foreign currency. However, some studies have costed these staff using local physician wages, arguing that, if the expatriate staff leave, they would be replaced by local physicians. The validity of this approach depends on the purpose of the costing analysis. If the aim is to project future budget/resource needs after the expatriates leave, then using local wage rates is appropriate. However, if the goal is to estimate current unit costs, local wages may understate the true cost of resources used depending on the currency rate and differentials between expatriate and local wages. Thus, the rationale behind the costing analysis will drive which measure is most appropriate.

In some cases, individuals may be employed and paid by more than one hospital. In each case, the proportion of their time spent in each hospital must be determined and applied accordingly. For example, if an employee spends four days working in your hospital and one day a week elsewhere, then you should be only paying 80% of his/her salary and the other facility paying the remaining 20%. The same rationale should be applied to fringe benefits.

Fringe Benefits: In principle, fringe benefits (e.g. health care insurance, vacation and sick pay, dental care, etc.) received by personnel as part of their employment should be included as part of total payroll costs. This is true whether these benefits are paid by the hospital and/or public sector funds managed by the Ministry of Health. Examples of such benefits are "gratuities" to physicians (the St. Lucia study) and employees' share of hospital fees or revenues (the Niger study).

To obtain a full, accurate picture of personnel costs of a hospital, one may need to know not only the cost of paid salaries and fringe benefits but, for planning purposes, may be interested in "inkind costs" (like unpaid work time or volunteer time). In a hospital study in Colombia, Robertson and colleagues measured unpaid work time along with fringe benefits and determined that both accounted for 40% of true personnel costs (or 30% of total direct costs). They measured unpaid work time by using outside observers to monitor staff activities and record time-study measurements for each employee. An example of unpaid work is time spent treating patients beyond normal clinic hours because of physician or nursing inefficiencies, overbookings and/or missed appointments. By not including unpaid labor when determining levels of productivity or efficiency, program managers or planners may make an erroneous conclusion.

Donated Items: Typically, when materials and equipment have been provided by foreign donors, they will not appear in hospital spending records. However, since the hospital is using these donated items, they should be included in calculations of hospital unit cost. This is especially relevant for regional or national level health authorities responsible for comparing the performance of different hospitals. If the value of donated inputs is not included in the cost analysis, hospitals or wards with more donated items may appear more efficient than their peers, even though their actual efficiency may be the same. Such items can account for a substantial share of hospital resources. In a study in Niger, for example, donated drugs were 19% of total drug spending and donated food was 20% of total food spending.

The treatment of donated capital items is discussed later. In this section we consider donated recurrent items, that is, those used up within the analysis period. Examples of these would be bandages, and syringes. The correct costing procedure is to prepare a list of these items and find out the replacement cost of each (i.e., what it now would cost to purchase each).

It is worth explaining the reasons to cost donated items, since in some situations, they may not apply. First, donated items may have an "opportunity cost," that is, one may want to consider how productive they would be if transferred to a different ward or hospital than the one where they currently happen to be used.

This issue is less relevant if the donation cannot be transferred (e.g. due to restrictions imposed by the donor) *and* the ministry cannot reallocate funds toward hospitals which receive fewer donations (e.g. due to 'maintenance of effort' restrictions imposed by donors). The second reason to cost donated items is that, at some point, donations may dry up or a long-lived donated good may need replacing. The hospital needs to anticipate these possibilities. As mentioned previously, the third reason is to avoid penalizing hospitals which look inefficient compared to others merely because they receive fewer donations.

Ministry of Health Spending

In many countries, the Ministry of Health pays directly for some resources used by hospitals, for example, stationery, vehicle maintenance and even salaries. This arrangement poses no special problem if the ministry keeps records on how funding was allocated among hospitals. When this is the case, you need only to add allocations to the appropriate expenditure line items. However, sometimes the ministry cannot determine specific spending levels by hospital. In this case, you will need to estimate the allocated amounts by line item yourself, preferably in consultation with officials at your hospital and the ministry. For example, in Tuvalu, most spending on the single hospital came from the ministry's budget and was not distinguished from spending on other health centres. The study authors estimated the hospital's share for each line item after discussion with those involved. These discussions suggested that, for example, the hospital accounted for 100% of lab costs, 90% of electricity, and 80% of medical supplies. These suggested percentages were applied to the national expenditure data, and the resulting figures were assigned to the hospital.

Drugs

Sometimes spending data on drugs and other consumable medical supplies are not available from the hospital's own accounts or those of the central ministry. For example, in some countries, drugs are purchased by a centralized government agency, which then supplies the drugs to hospitals without this appearing in the Ministry of Health or hospital budget. In such cases, it is necessary to access the agency's records, and determine the value of drugs shipped to the hospital(s) of interest. Sometimes (as in the Papua New Guinea study) the central agency can provide a printout of the value of shipments. Othertimes, only quantities are reported, in which case the value of the drugs can be computed by obtaining the price paid for each drug item and multiplying this figure by the respective quantity.

If the agency recorded which departments within each hospital ordered or received the drugs, this information is important for later stages of the cost analysis, and should be included in any transfer of data.

The large volume of drug data may make it impractical to analyze a full year experience. In some studies, consultants analyzed a sample of pharmacy records rather than a full year of data. In fact, to estimate one year's use, the St. Lucia study used a two-month sample of pharmacy requisitions from the Central Medical Stores. If this approach is taken, one should try to sample various points in the year to account for seasonal variations in drug utilization.

As in the case of Mills' Malawi study, the hospital pharmacy can have information on drug deliveries to each ward but may not know the value or price of the drugs. If this is due to drugs being paid by a centralized government agency, then one can ask the agency the price it pays for each of the drugs concerned and evaluate drug consumption using those prices.

Fuel

If actual records of spending on fuel are not available, it may be possible to estimate spending indirectly. Some hospitals keep logbooks for personnel to record vehicle mileage for all trips. By estimating the number of miles-per-gallon performance, one can convert these mileage totals into estimates of total petrol (gasoline) consumed over a given period. In turn, petrol spending can be estimated by valuing the petrol consumption at the local retail price per gallon or litre. Similarly, spending figures may be unavailable for generators and other hospital equipment. As in the case of the WHO Gambia study, spending can be estimated using information about how often the equipment is used, the rate at which it consumes fuel, and the price per unit of fuel.

Maintenance

In some countries, personnel who maintain public hospitals are employed by the ministry of health rather than the individual hospital. Ignoring this practice might lead one to understate the true cost of operating the hospital. As with other centrally supplied inputs (such as drugs), the question is whether the central agency can report how much service it provided to each hospital. If not, one must devise a rule to allocate some portion of the central maintenance budget to each hospital being studied. The simplest way would be to assume that the hospital's share of maintenance costs is proportional to its area (square feet or metres). A more accurate approach might then be to weigh older hospitals more heavily, assuming they need more intensive maintenance.

Spending from User Fee Revenue

A Common Component of Many Cost Recovery programs is to allow the hospital to retain a portion of fees charged for its discretion. For example, in the Jamaican hospitals studied by Kutzin, hospitals were allowed to keep 50% of revenues generated. Spending of retained revenues may be hard to measure especially if financial controls are poor. Yet, it is important to try, given the growing importance of this revenue source in many poor countries.

In some countries the amount of revenues retained (or costs recovered) is not welldocumented.

If this is the case, one can estimate retained revenues by applying the fee schedule to available utilization data. For example, if the hospital charges 10 francs per outpatient visit and 50 francs per inpatient day, and provided 1000 outpatient visits and 1000 inpatient days on a monthly basis, then the total fee revenue for that time period would be 60,000 francs ([10 x 1000] + [50 x 1000]). If some patients received free care due to their inability to pay or incomplete collection, total cost recovery would be overstated if not taken into account.

Having estimated total cost recovery, one can determine how the money was spent by line item or cost centre. Even if hospital records do not indicate uses of fee revenues, interviews with staff may shed light on this question. For example, through staff interviews, Kutzin concluded that the Jamaican hospitals were spending much of their revenue fees on "breakdown" maintenance.

A further complication exists in hospitals where staff are practicing 'unofficial' cost recovery without transmitting the proceeds to the hospital accounts. Ojo and colleagues estimated these amounts to be substantial in the Sierra Leone hospitals which they studied. Even if one can measure these amounts, their treatment depends on how one thinks they are being spent and the purpose of the analysis.

If staff are spending the money to buy supplies, then these are costs of the hospital and should be included in a cost analysis (if measurable). If the unofficial fees are being treated as private income by staff, and spent outside the hospital, then they should not be included in a hospital cost analysis. On the other hand, the amounts collected may be relevant to a cost recovery analysis, as they indicate patients' willingness to pay which might be better tapped by the hospital itself.

Delayed Payments

As in Conventional Accounting Analysis, Cost Measures may be Misstated when services are paid in a different accounting period from when they are used. The Jamaica study by Kutzin found large fluctuations in utility payments which did not reflect real resource use even within a fiscal year. This occurred because some hospitals were able to delay payment for months, then later make large settlements. The study author corrected for this by using actual kilowatt-hours when available, and otherwise using hospitals' budget requests for utilities. Without the correction, the same facility would have shown variations over time in calculated unit cost which would be difficult to explain.

Capital Items

Capital assets are assets having an economic useful life exceeding one year and not acquired primarily for resale. A unit cost analysis which ignores capital is essentially assuming that the present physical assets will be available forever. In reality, assets are being worn down by the hospital's daily activities, and this depreciation is an expense.

Unlike drug purchases or salaries, depreciation is not an expenditure, it does not require an actual cost outlay. However, depreciation may be hard to measure, if certain information is not available (such as purchase price and the useful life of its equipment). If this is the case, then determining the depreciation expense becomes more sensitive to the analyst's assumptions.

For the present analysis, we are not necessarily trying to compute a "depreciation allowance," or how much to save up for equipment replacement. Rather, the aim is to estimate the opportunity cost of the capital being used up, in a way that is consistent across periods.

Reflecting this, the methodology we present here differs somewhat from more accounting-based approaches with which you may be familiar.

If one decides to measure the cost of eventually replacing capital, then several questions must be answered for each asset:

What is the Asset's Total Life?

A typical assumption for a building is a total life of 30 years. Other studies have assumed that beds and furniture last 10 years, and vehicles last five years. The assumption matters most for items with a large share of cost, for example, buildings, vehicles and major medical equipment.

What will be the Cost of Replacing it at the End of the Year?

Financial accounts often calculate depreciation based on an asset's original purchase price ('historic cost'). However, if there is inflation (as in most countries), historic cost will understate the amount required to replace a given asset. Replacement cost is the more relevant measure for those planning resource use.

From this viewpoint, the original purchase cost is really only useful as a starting point for figuring out the cost of replacing the asset. Of course, even the original cost may not be available, if it was purchased by a donor or the ministry of health. Assuming some estimate of original cost is made, this must then be updated to this year and each future year in which replacement could occur. In other words, one must forecast the inflation which is likely to occur from now until the year of replacement.

Estimates of local inflation are often available from governments or aid agencies for a number of years ahead, but become increasingly unavailable (and unreliable) beyond five years.

If the replacement must be paid with foreign currency, one should also predict how the cost of foreign currency (i.e., the exchange rate) will change over the period in question. Sometimes exchange rate forecasts are available from the central bank, or otherwise one can extrapolate from recent experience. In the Gambia study, the authors assumed an annual exchange rate deterioration of 27%.

What Interest Rate should be Applied to Money Saved now for Future Replacement?

Calculations of a 'capital cost' typically apply some kind of interest rate, based on the local return to a savings account. This is often justified by imagining that the hospital is saving up to replace its equipment, and can deposit the savings in an interest-bearing account. This approach has been criticized by Carrin and others, as unrealistic in many developing countries where public hospitals lack authority to save in this way.

The method we propose here continues to use the real (inflation free) interest rate, but we justify it by imagining that the hospital could rent medical equipment instead of buying it. To find the maximum rental payment the hospital should be willing to make, one would use this same approach (assuming perfect capital markets).

Finally, given the uncertainty associated with measurements of capital costs, it may be advisable to present two sets of results, one including capital cost and one excluding it. This approach was taken by Ojo and colleagues in Sierra Leone. Their results show that including capital costs substantially increases unit costs on inpatient wards (30 to 50%) but has little effect on unit costs of the operating room. This appears to be because the wards had more valuable equipment and, in most cases, more floor space than the operating theatre.

In general, we suggest using a real interest rate of 3%. This rate has been found in many industrialized and developing economies. As this rate was used in a comprehensive set of cost effectiveness studies for the health sector (Jamison et al 1993) its use makes hospital costing consistent with the international literature.

Assignment of Inputs to Cost Centres

At this point, you have presumably gathered information about the hospital's total costs, whatever the source of payment. This information alone may provide useful insights even before you start computing unit costs: for example, in identifying which line items account for most of cost and whether this is changing over time. However, to compute unit costs one must proceed to the next step: assigning costs from each line item to the relevant cost centres.

Some inputs can be assigned directly to certain cost centres. For example, if 'kitchen' is a cost centre, then the line item 'food' could all be assigned to that cost centre. More often, inputs are used by several cost centres, and the analyst must seek to assign spending for an input across those centres.

Correct assignment is most important for those inputs which account for a larger share of costs, such as staff time and drugs.

Staff Time

A variety of methods have been used to assign staff time among cost centres, ranging from simple (using administrative data) to elaborate (direct measurement).

Administrative data: Many hospitals have duty rosters showing which staff are assigned to which departments. Since many staff typically work in only one department, the roster can be used to allocate these staff. For the remainder who work in multiple departments, you can interview them individually, which may be time-consuming if they are numerous. Alternatively, you could ask their manager how many hours they work in each department, and prorate their salary (and fringe benefits) accordingly.

Direct measurement: The Dominican Republic study by Lewis and colleagues used the most comprehensive approach to allocating staff time. They employed data collectors who followed medical staff over a period of weeks and recorded the time spent with each patient. This was supplemented by interviews with patients. The study authors found that physicians only worked 12% of the time for which they were paid. This is an example of how the process of cost analysis can generate important information, even without computing unit costs. The information they gained was that the hospital was paying for labor it did not obtain.)

Comparison of approaches: The direct measurement approach has the advantage of giving direct information about the sources of inefficiency, where other approaches merely identify to which cost centre expenditures should be assigned. The disadvantage of the direct-measurement approach is the high cost of implementing it, at least in the way defined by Lewis and colleagues. Analysts may want to consider a more limited implementation, perhaps in the second phase of a hospital cost study after getting other systems working. The simplest method is to examine duty rosters for staff (if available), and allocate their time and associated salaries and fringes accordingly.

Excluded Activities

At some hospitals, certain activities generate costs which need to be excluded from the unit cost computation. There are several possible reasons for such exclusion:

Non-patient care: The prime example is teaching. Suppose you plan to compare unit costs between some hospitals which do a lot of teaching and others which do not. The teaching hospitals will naturally appear to have higher costs, even if they provide patient care very efficiently. In this situation, it is desirable to identify and exclude teaching costs to the extent possible. Some costs may be identifiable using job rosters which identify how many hours were spent teaching. However, teaching and patient care often occur simultaneously. Robertson and colleagues developed an approach to this in their Colombia study, which tracked physicians with time-and-motion methods.

When care was being provided by a resident, the resident's time was charged to patient care while the supervisor's time was charged to teaching. When the resident and physician-supervisor conferred after seeing a patient, the time of both was charged to teaching.

Not under hospital control: Sometimes the central government operates some directly controlled programs on the hospital premises: for example, immunization campaigns. If these programs are not under the hospital's control, it would be unreasonable to include them in the hospital's unit costs. In both cases, the excluded activities should be treated as final cost centres, in the sense that overhead will be allocated to them, and they will not be reallocated to other centres. However, unit costs will not be computed for them (unless you are interested and can identify outputs to measure).

Drugs

Drugs usually account for a substantial share of hospital resources, so it matters how their costs are treated in your analysis.

If you are hoping to compute a unit cost per prescription, then you will definitely need to create a separate cost centre for drugs (say, 'pharmacy'). If you are not treating drugs as an 'output', then you can choose between two approaches:

- Create a separate 'pharmacy' cost centre but allocate its costs to final cost centres *during* the stepdown process
- Assign drug costs to the cost centres (intermediate and final) *before* the step-down process.

Each approach has different advantages. The first approach is simpler, in that pharmacy costs will eventually be allocated based on a single statistic (e.g., each ward's share of prescriptions written).

The second approach has value if you have better information, and know you can do better than allocating drugs based on a single statistic. For example, if you have data on the value of each department's actual drug purchases, you could assign the currency amounts to each department at this stage. However, against this, there is a managerial issue: the pharmacy is usually a separate hospital department run by a manager or responsible person, who should be able to track (and account for) use of the resources provided.

The pharmacy manager will be better able to manage resources if the pharmacy is treated as a separate cost centre. In addition, identifying Pharmacy as a separate cost centre in all hospitals would help regional and national managers to monitor and compare the relative performance of pharmacy departments in different hospitals. Therefore, we would regard this as the preferred option, barring exceptional circumstances.

Allocation of all Costs to Final Cost Centres

The next step is to reallocate all indirect costs to the final cost centres. In this way, the unit cost will include overhead costs incurred in producing an admission, day or visit, not just direct costs. Indirect costs will include all costs which could not be allocated directly to final cost centres at an earlier stage. In some hospitals, this will only comprise services such as administration and laundry. In others, intermediate services such as pharmacy and radiology may also need allocating at this point, with little or no information about how much of their workload was generated by each of the medical departments.

Allocation Basis

Where each department's use of an indirect cost centre is unknown, one must devise some rule to allocate the indirect costs across departments. The rule is called an 'allocation basis', and is intended to reflect whatever factors determine each department's use of the indirect (i.e., overhead, intermediate, or general) cost centre. These factors may differ depending on the centre. For example, most studies allocate laundry costs among wards based on the percentage distribution of total patient-days in each ward, since patients who stay longer use more laundry services. On the other hand, cleaning services are often allocated according to each department's floor area, since more spacious departments cost more to clean. (Of course, this may involve measuring the floor area of each department if such information is not readily available from sources such as building plans).

Knowledge of your own hospital may lead you to devise an allocation basis which predicts costs accurately, even if it has not been used elsewhere. For example, Weaver et al., the authors of the Niger study, decided that the number of air-conditioning units would be a good predictor of water and electricity costs, so they used that basis to allocate utility costs across wards (i.e., percentage distribution of air-conditioning units). They also learned that patients in private wards received were served better food, so that it would be incorrect to allocate kitchen cost simply based on the number of bed-days. Instead, they used a weighting scheme in which one day in a private room was equivalent to several days in the general ward. This example shows the importance of the judgment and creativity that the person doing costing may bring from specific knowledge of the hospital or the local situation.

List of Cost Centres in Lesotho Study

Direct Patient Care

1. Adult medical/surgical wards
2. Theater

3. Obstetric wards
4. Pediatric wards
5. Satellite clinics
6. Public health
7. Dental
8. Casualty
9. Clinics
10. Nursing.

Ancillary Clinical Services

11. Pharmacy
12. Laboratory and blood bank
13. Radiology
14. Physiotherapy
15. Orthopedic workshop.

Support Services

16. Sterile supply
17. Maintenance
18. Security
19. Food service
20. Laundry
21. Portering
22. Transport
23. Mortuary.

Administration

24. Medical records
25. Accounts
26. Personnel
27. Stores
28. Registry
29. All other administration.

Computing Unit Cost for Each Cost Centre

At this point you know the total costs that were incurred at each of the final cost centres.

What is the output of each centre, in days, discharges, lab tests etc.? This requires incorporating utilization data into the analysis.

In reality, you will have used the utilization data already by this point, for example in order to allocate laundry costs across wards in proportion to bed-days.

However, this is the point at which any problems with the utilization data become particularly important, because they directly alter the unit costs.

Several studies encountered problems with utilization data. In some cases, the number of admissions seemed accurate, but admission and discharge dates had not been carefully recorded, causing measurement of bed-days to be inaccurate.

Correct measurement of bed-days requires that staff count how many beds are occupied in every ward, every 24 hours at the same time of day. The authors of the Lesotho study recommend that this should be done at midnight. A recent report on a Zambian hospital gives details on one way to conduct a bed census (Buve and Foster,1995).

Once you have obtained the utilization data, the unit cost can be computed. For each of the final cost centres, divide its fully allocated cost by its units of service.

Reporting Results

At this point it is important to remind yourself and any readers what items are and are not included in the unit costs you have calculated. For example, your unit cost does not include drugs and x-rays unless you specifically allocated the costs of those services to other final cost centres, during steps 5 and 6.

Similarly, if you are not reporting outputs for certain final cost centres (e.g. teaching, public health clinic) then it is worth saying so in a footnote. Otherwise, readers may assume these centres' costs have been allocated to the services for which you do report unit costs.

Hospital Revenues

The revenue generated by a hospital, expressed as a proportion of its costs, is the product of three factors: the fee level (average fee as a proportion of average unit cost), the proportion of services which are paying (not exempted), and the collection efficiency (proportion of fees owed which are actually collected and remitted to the hospital's account). Generally, only a share of patients are actually charged the set fee, with the remaining ones being exempted due to poverty or other privileged categories (e.g. school children, or disabled war veterans).

The first two factors are policy variables set by the hospital. A high degree of acceptability and a high degree of affordability for the service favor setting these percentages high, while a high level of costeffectiveness and a high elasticity of demand favor lower fees and proportion paying. The last factor is a measure of administrative capacity. The efficiency of collection is greatest when only a few providers can dispense a given service in a limited location, and when the service is generally provided on an elective basis.

The "current situation" represents the authors' impression of fee collections in government hospitals in Bangladesh and Zimbabwe, where the manual was discussed in workshops. The fee level is currently low overall because fees for inpatient services and drugs generally cover only a small share of the costs involved, and these costs represent the majority of the operating costs of the country's hospitals. The proportion paying is also low because of broadly defined policies of indigence. As hospitals do not retain the fees they collect, they have every reason to be generous in interpreting the need for an exemption.

Finally, the collection factor reflects the absence of specific programs to enhance collection.

In Jamaica, where a comparable collection rate previously existed, efforts of the Health

Sector Initiatives Program substantially increased revenues. There, hospitals were given the liquidity and flexibility of spending their revenues, even though their government subsidies were often reduced as revenues rose. Collectors were trained, building modifications were made if needed to create a cashier's window, and additional positions were created to ensure that cashiers were on duty during evenings and weekends, in addition to normal government hours.

The "high fee" scenario below shows what would happen if nominal prices were set with no subsidies (i.e., 100% of costs). With only a moderate proportion of patients asked to pay (50%), and a low level of collections (40%), the overall level of cost recovery is 30%. By contrast, the same revenue is raised with a more moderate level of fees (15% lower on average), the same level of exemptions (50%), but better collections (70% enforcement). In some hospitals, "leakage" in collections occurs between the patient and the hospital account. While the patient may pay an "informal" fee, it may be retained by a gatekeeper, personal attendant, aide, nurse, physician, or deposited in a location other than the official hospital account. To improve collection, administrators may consider establishing policies to ensure that at least part of official fees are retained by the hospital that collects them and used to visibly benefit the institution, the patients, and the staff.

Estimating Volumes in a Hospital System

Projections from Very Limited Data. The most limited situation occurs when only two very limited types of data are available for an individual hospital or a system of similar hospitals: the total operating costs and some measure(s) of size or activities. The preferable measure of size or activities is the number of services performed during a given period (such as the last year). A usable proxy, however, is the number of beds.

Shepard and Gonzales (1982) used this approximation to project the cost impact of a major expansion in hospitals underway in Honduras from 1980 to 1983. With data on the numbers of beds and recurrent costs for general public hospitals, they calculated that the annual operating cost per bed had grown at a 6.9% real annual rate of growth from 1976 to 1980 because of increasing intensity of services (or simply because of increasing budget allocations).

They used this trend to project the future cost per bed. They multiplied it times the projected future number of beds (computed by adding beds under construction/planned to current bed capacity). To the consternation of financial officials, the results proved realistic. With the construction and planning processes well underway, the Ministry and donors added the beds essentially as scheduled. Financial constraints delayed the opening of several hospitals, however, until years after they were completed. Similar approaches could be applied to an individual hospital, or to various types of hospital systems, such as:

- all government district hospitals in a given region, or in the country as a whole;
- all provincial hospitals in the country;
- all multi-purpose referral or teaching hospitals in a given region, or in the country as a whole;
- all specialty hospitals with a given purpose, such as mental health, tuberculosis.

Estimating Costs From Relative Values. A more accurate approach is feasible if data are available on the volume of services produced (activities) for a hospital over a defined period (generally one year), as well as on the annual operating costs. This approach differs from that in the preceding chapter, however, because it does not require operating costs to be assigned to individual departments or cost centres. Deriving unit costs from these data entails the following five steps.

Identify the Output-producing Centres

As in the preceding chapter, the question is: for which services will unit costs be computed? This choice depends primarily on the level of detail for which activity data are available. For most hospitals, data are available on at least the aggregate number of ambulatory visits and the aggregate number of inpatient bed-days per year. In this case, one can estimate total cost of inpatient versus outpatient care and the unit costs of a bed day and ambulatory visit. In some cases, the number of bed-days is reported by clinical department or ward (e.g., medicine, surgery, and maternity). In that case, one can estimate the unit costs per bed-day by ward.

Define Units of Output

For each patient ca.e cost centre, one must define a unit of output. Within each cost centre, the unit of output must be readily counted and reasonably homogeneous. In most cases, inpatient services are best expressed in terms of days, and ambulatory services in terms of visits.

Inpatient admissions represents an alternative, though less homogeneous, measure. Costs will then be expressed in terms of per day or per visit. If data are also available on admissions as well as patient days, this will allow for a calculation of average length of stay (ALOS). Average cost per admission could then be calculated by multiplying the estimate of average cost per day times

ALOS

Define the data period: Data can be analyzed on a per-year, per-quarter or other basis. The crucial issue is to make sure that the same time period applies both to your aggregate cost figure and your utilization data.

Identify the full Costs of the Facility

Financial statements for the hospital may be a useful starting point, although as previously noted they may understate cost. Where possible you should try to add in costs of resources used by the hospital but paid for by others, e.g.

- donated items
- drugs purchased by a central state agency
- employees' time paid for out of other budgets.

Obtain External Data on Relative Costliness of Services

To implement this approach, you will need estimates of the relative costliness of different types of care. These are rules of thumb, such as:

- One day of inpatient care costs three times as much as one outpatient visit.
- One surgical admission costs 10% more than the average inpatient admission overall.

We call these data 'external' because they will have to come from outside your hospital.

Possible sources for these estimates could include:

- Other hospitals in your country for which step-down cost accounting studies have been done
- Judgment of clinical experts or hospital staff on the relative amounts of resources used for the different services
- Studies from other countries you are familiar with
- However, you will generate more useful information if you use estimates from hospitals which are similar to your own (e.g. in the same country, same level of hospital).

Allocation of a Budget among Hospitals

Bed-day equivalents provide a useful statistic to allocate a central budget equitably among public hospitals. If this statistic were the only one used, then each hospital would receive a budget proportional to its share of total bed-day equivalents. That is, if a hospital generated 10% of the country's bed-day equivalents in the latest year with full data, it would be awarded 10% of the country's hospital budget next year. This statistic is one of the terms in the formula used by the Zimbabwe Ministry of Health to allocate funds to its central hospitals and provinces.

While not perfect, this type of system has several advantages. It is more objective and rational than the allocations based on past budgets and political influence seemingly practiced in some countries. It rewards productivity and efficiency, so each hospital receives the same budget per inpatient day and per outpatient visit. By contrast, budgets based on historical costs perpetuate, and may even encourage, overspending and inefficiency.

Limitations of a system based on bed day equivalents are its exclusion of several important factors, and its possible perverse incentives. A system based solely on bed-day equivalents would fail to account for needs for preventive and promotive services (which are not measured by inpatient and outpatient services), for differences in the sophistication of services, for other factors affecting the costs of services (e.g., distance and scale), for varying abilities of hospitals to raise revenue (based on the capacity to pay of the populations they serve), and for the time and central support required for a hospital to adjust to a different budget (i.e., to transfer personnel in or out, trim costs responsibly, or use additional funds productively). Perverse incentives can arise because such a system would reward provider-induced utilization (i.e., excessive admissions, lengths of say, or follow up visits to boost activity statistics).

These limitations can be addressed by incorporating other factors in the allocation formula, and using a blended formula based on a combination of bed-day equivalents and historic budgets. The Zimbabwe Ministry of Health has addressed many of these concerns by using 13 parameters (including bed-day equivalents) in its allocations of resources. Other factors include population (a proxy for the needs of preventive services), area (a proxy for distance among facilities), numbers of health facilities and of rural health clinics (measures of scale), total beds, number of vehicles, dental ratios, laboratory units (all measures of sophistication), staff salaries and allowances (measures of past budgets), and outpatient attendances, patient days, and occupied beds (all additional measures of volume of activities). Each hospital's allocation is a weighted average of its share of the national total on each of these factors. While the Zimbabwe system does not explicitly incorporate relative income of catchment populations in its formula, this term could be included in a final adjustment allowed by its system—"manual moderation taking into account practical factors" (Zimbabwe Ministry of Health, 1994).

Applications to Improve Hospital Efficiency

Overall efficiency. The manager of a hospital system should calculate the unit costs of final outputs for each of the hospitals in the system, and compare the results for the same unit of service in hospitals of the same type (e.g., district, provincial, and referral). For example, costs per patient-day and per outpatient visit can be compared.

For hospitals of comparable sophistication and quality, a low cost per patient-day is an indication of good efficiency, while a high cost per patient-day may suggest poor efficiency. A manager will first want to examine the data to rule out three spurious factors. First, if unit costs are excessively high in one hospital, resources may have been over-allocated to that hospital and under-allocated to another. For example, suppose two institutions share some important service, such as a pharmacy but all, or almost all, the cost were allocated to just one institution. Then the costs of that institution would be inappropriately high, while those of the other would be inordinately low. The manager should examine the unit costs of hospitals that might share services to see if they are inordinately low. If so, he or she should consider revising the basis of allocating the shared resource to see if results change substantially.

Second, the share of resources allocated to a particular service may have been inappropriately high. For example, if a hospital's cost for an outpatient visit were high, perhaps an excessive share of personnel or pharmacy costs was allocated to that service. To determine whether this spurious factor is responsible, the manager should examine possible reallocations of that resource. A service which represents a small share of a hospital's total costs is especially prone to errors in allocation. A small absolute difference in allocation will then make a big relative change in unit costs. For example, suppose a manager were unsure whether an emergency (casualty) ward represented 5 or 10 percent of hospital personnel. The total personnel costs, and thus the unit personnel costs, will be twice as high under the 10 percent allocation. For a large service, however, a 5 percentage point difference is much less crucial. The difference of 5 percentage points between, say a 50 versus a 55 percent share of personnel for medical/surgical inpatient stays would change unit costs by only a tenth. If unit costs for a given hospital tend to be very high for some services and very low for others, then it is possible that the basis of allocation is in appropriate. On the other hand, if a hospital's unit cost is consistently above average for different services, then that hospital is probably less efficient.

Third, an especially low unit cost may indicate that important resources are not being counted, or an estimate for a resource is particularly high. Results from Connaught Hospital in Sierra Leone may indicate this type of result. Many drugs and supplies were not bought officially through the hospital pharmacy (which had limited stock), but were purchased by patients, either through commercial pharmacies in the city, or through semi-formal drug sales at the hospital pharmacy. A knowledge of the hospital's operations facilitates these interpretations.

Once these spurious factors have been ruled out, it is instructive to examine the most efficient hospitals. Characteristics worth noting are: occupancy rate, staffing per bed, and per patient day, the proportion of staff at each of several levels of skill:

- doctor (includes dentists and licenses pharmacists)
- other health and management professional (include nurses, technicians, therapists, administrators)
- non-professional (driver, aides, housekeepers).

The standards of the most efficient hospital are often worth emulating.

Analysis of intermediate cost centres. A cost analysis generates the breakdown of total and unit costs by cost centres. Managers can judge these results against policy norms of how they think money *ought* to be spent, as well as against the positive data of how money *actually* was spent in other times and hospitals.

For example, the Sierra Leone study (Ojo et al., 1995) reported that food for patients represented the majority of costs in the country's referral hospital. As food is a less essential part of the process of hospital treatment than professional advice and medicines, it does not deserve a larger share of hospital budgets. Thus, anomalous allocation of resources prompts examining why food costs are so high. Both data anomalies and real managerial characteristics need to be examined. In Sierra Leone, Ojo et al. (1995) reported that the cost of food (the equivalent of $5 per patient per day) was based on an estimate of the value of food given by an international donor. Either the estimate was high, or the food given was worth exceptionally high amounts.

Similarly, it is possible to compare results of a specific cost centre across hospitals. We suggest examining the cost of this cost centre through three ratios: (1) overall costliness: per patient day, (2) intensity: units of service per patient day, and (3) unit costs:

cost per unit of service. The first ratio measures the overall resources used by a cost centre, combining both utilization and costliness of that cost centre. The second ratio is derived by measuring the allocated cost of an intermediate cost centre divided by the total units of service. The third ratio is derived by dividing the total cost of the intermediate cost centre by its allocation statistic. The three ratios are related by the mathematical identity: (1) = (2) x (3). This relationship allows the consistency of the data to be verified. An important advantage of this decomposition is that different officials are often responsible for different ratios. While responsibility is shared for the cleaning cost per bed day, the service intensity largely reflects choices in partitioning space among services, while the unit costs reflects decisions of the person responsible for the cleaning service.

Hospital's Role in the Health System

One of the principles of health planning is that patient should be treated in the least complex and least costly type of health facility which is adequate for their needs. This rule would generally ensure that patients are treated more conveniently, at lesser cost to the family (because they save travel expenses), and often at lower cost to the health system (as lower level facilities are thought to be less costly). Unit cost analysis allows the economic rationale behind this policy to be examined. For example, are tertiary hospitals really producing care more expensively than lower-level hospitals? If the tertiary hospitals have unit costs three times higher for the same services, should their fees also be three times higher? As with other "real world" policies, cost alone is not a sufficient factor. Important dimensions of quality need examination. Quality entails not only the excellence of the staff, the depth of their training, and the sophistication of their infrastructure. Promptness and courtesy of service are also highly valued by patients. Nevertheless, there are potential economic gains from a more rigorous management of referral procedures.

Disease Specific Costs

Among adults, the prevalence of HIV infection in developing countries (1.5%) is 13 times as high as in industrialized countries

(0.12%) (Mann and Tarantola, 1996). To better plan responses for prevention and control both donors and national governments needed data on current levels of health expenditures related to HIV/AIDS, their allocations and sources. Hospital costs represent a critical component of overall costs. In a study sponsored by the World Bank, the European Commission, and UNAIDS, Shepard (1996) selected five countries of varying economic levels for case studies. Only the one with the highest per capita GDP, Brazil, had existing data on hospital expenditures for AIDS. These were derived from reimbursements through its government run social security system.

For the other countries, several sources of data needed to be assembled. The Cote d'Ivoire (CI), a country of 14.3 million persons severely affected by this condition, illustrates this process (Shepard, 1996). Estimates for the CI were based on both objective data and Delphi estimates by AIDS experts from government, voluntary hospitals, and traditional medicine (Kone et al., 1996).

First, the overall number of AIDS patients was derived from reported cases and expanded for underreporting. Second, the experts classified the estimated annual number of new HIV/AIDS clinical cases into five groups based on the expected type and amount of care that they typically received. Third, the length of stay and setting for each group was based on clinical data. Fourth, unit costs in each type of hospital were based on available unit cost studies, derived from step-down analyses or relative value approaches. For example, patients with private insurance coverage were estimated to receive care at private clinics, costing on average 52,500 West African Francs (F CFA, equivalent to US $105) per day. At the other extreme, the hospitals used by rural patients (largely public, district hospitals) cost 5,000 F CFA ($10) per day. Finally, totals were computed.

Cost Effectiveness Analysis: Disease Control Approaches

As a final application, cost analysis can help policy makers compare alternative approaches to controlling a given disease.

First, it can allow simple comparisons such as ambulatory versus inpatient surgery. A Colombian study, for example, found that the ambulatory form of surgery for repair of an uncomplicated hernia cost only a quarter as much as the inpatient form (Shepard et al., 1993).

Finally, cost analysis can allow approaches based on very different approaches to be compared. For example, for two important health problems in many tropical countries, prevention is difficult. Respiratory infections are airborne. Dengue viruses are carried by mosquitoes that breed quickly, even when spraying has reduced their number. Cost-effectiveness analysis of control programs for both diseases showed that except for vaccination, case management was generally the most cost-effective control procedure. An analysis of hospital costs helped derive the costs of the case management approach.

Hospital financing: User Fees

Cost analysis is an important ingredient in setting levels of user fees.

In practice, user fees are guided by additional considerations. Currently, hospital services in the public sector are heavily subsidized in almost every country. User fees commonly recover only a tenth of hospital costs.

Governments can, and often should, continue to subsidize care at public hospitals.

Nevertheless, the calculation of unit costs allows that subsidy to be allocated more rationally.

Principles of social welfare policy indicate that subsidies should be granted under the following conditions. First, if the consumers of a service are poor, so that the subsidy is a kind of in-kind income transfer to them. Second, if the service is a merit good or public good, so that the government wants consumers to use it. Many primary care services, and especially immunization, fit this second criterion.

The above analysis suggests that there is little rationale for subsidizing amenity services primarily consumed by the well off. Analysis of unit costs will indicate how much they should be charged over the long run.

Hospital Financing: Insurance. A number of developing countries are considering, or starting to implement systems of national health insurance. For example, Colombia passed a health reform law in 1994. Trinidad and Tobago completed a major study, and Ivory Coast is planning pilot programs. Typically, these systems entail payment by the insurance system to the provider of care (a hospital or doctor). Unit cost analysis allows an appropriate rate of payment to be developed.

In countries which allow multiple insurers to emerge, there is some risk that each insurer will try to pay less than its share of the hospital's overhead. This has been a problem in the United States, where some insurers have allegedly 'shifted costs' onto others by setting low payment rates. Measuring unit costs can help sort out these issues, by distinguishing direct costs of an admission (to be paid by the insurer responsible) from overhead costs (to be prorated across insurers). In principle, the government could prevent cost-shifting by requiring every insurer to pay the unit cost of a discharge. In practice, this may be undesirable, as hospitals might lose their incentive to restrain overhead costs .

Demonstrating Excellence in Practice -based Research for Public Health

In 1853, physician John Snow provided one of public health's first models of practice-based research. His epidemiologic research that led to removing the handle from the communal Broad Street pump to prevent further cholera infections is a landmark example of practicebased research for all who confront today's most complex public health problems.

Demonstrating Excellence in Practice-Based Research for Public Health is intended for those who produce, participate in, and use practice-based research. This includes academic researchers community-based organizations and professionals, and interested members of the community. The purpose of this document is to demonstrate the contributions and benefits of conducting inter-, multi-, and transdisciplinary research for community health improvement. [A *community* is an aspect of collective and individual identity characterized by a sense of identification and emotional connection to other members. Further, this document serves as a resource for academic public health institutions in fulfilling their social responsibility to their communities, community partner organizations, and health departments, such as providing technical assistance to improve services delivered by health departments and other public health organizations.

Eight Characteristics of Practice-Based Research for Public Health

1. Scholarly. Practice-based research is manifested in Boyer's four dimensions of public health scholarship: discovery, application, integration, and teaching.
2. Rigorous. Practice-based research is evidence-based and is subject to standards of rigor and peer-evaluation.
3. Practical. Practice-based research addresses subject-matter derived from and/or relevant to public health practice and produces outputs that are useful to all of its participants and stakeholders.
4. Ecological. Practice-based research is conducted within an ecological paradigm that considers the health of individuals within biological, familial, social, environmental, and policy contexts.
5. Methodologically diverse. Practice-based research considers multiple (qualitative and quantitative) methodologies based on the nature of the public health problem; it recognizes the benefits of interdisciplinary, multidisciplinary, and transdisciplinary collaboration.
6. Collaborative. Practice-based research collaboratively involves practitioners, community organizations, and academic researchers to enhance knowledge and to improve practices toward ameliorating community health problems, improving the capacity of public health systems, and advancing the health status of populations.
7. Equitable. Practice-based research requires the equitable sharing of decision-making among public health practice agencies, community organizations, and academic researchers throughout the research process.

8. Translational. Practice-based research for public health emphasizes the means of converting and translating the latest research findings into timely and effective knowledge, tools, applications and policies that improve and advance the health of populations.

Historical Context for Practice-based Research

As public health continues to address the multiple determinants of health in the 21st century, the conduct and growth of practice-based research will increasingly depend on understanding an ecological paradigm of research, or the "interconnectedness of the biological, behavioural, physical and socio-environmental domains." Take, for example, the *Healthy People* goal to eliminate racial and ethnic health disparities. Given the multiple factors that impact population health, the steps toward achieving this goal call for multidisciplinary and transdisciplinary approaches within community settings using an ecological paradigm of research to improve public health policies and decision making.

Public health practitioners' reliance on evidence-based practices has evolved radically from the use of observational and bacteriological laboratory research in the 1880s. By the mid-20th century, when risk factors and prevention strategies for population-based diseases and injury were being identified and developed, community-based interventions were often implemented without the scientific backing required for clinical interventions. History informs what we do in public health and, in the latter part of the 20th century, progress in evidentiary practice-based research has grounded public health practice in science to improve population health through policy development and assurance activities such as: the development of community water fluoridation, detection of food sources in salmonella outbreaks, mass media campaigns to reduce tobacco use, the distribution of child auto safety seats, diabetes management programs, and mandatory school vaccinations.

In addition, research increasingly employs a wide-range of disciplines and various forms of inquiries that cross-fertilize epidemiology, sociology, policy, economics, and education, among others.

Stakeholders

The 2003 IOM Report, *The Future of the Public Health's in the 21st Century,* cites several recommendations that encourage proliferation of practice-based research environments, including the recommendation that research topics and funding be enhanced to address health problems at the levels of communities and populations.

Public and private organizations and agencies provide support for, and influence the progress of, practicebased research. They contribute to funding and to problem definition, suggest interventions, and incentivize interest and collaboration. The diversity of stakeholders provides exceptional opportunities to partner, dialogue, and leverage resources for research on difficult public health challenges.

Several government agencies have been engaged in promoting practice-based research and have committed resources to increase ecologically-based research and research training. For example, a major theme of the National Institutes of Health (NIH) strategic initiative, "Roadmap for Medical Research," is to create research teams that focus on interdisciplinary research and training. The population-focused research initiatives of the Centres for Disease Control and Prevention (CDC) reflect the characteristic that practice-based research is evidence-based and is subject to standards of rigor and peer evaluation, as exemplified in its funding of the Prevention Research Centres and the Injury Control and Research Centres. Furthermore, CDC-funded Centres for Public Health Preparedness and the Public.

Health Training Centre Network funded by the Health Resources and Services Administration (HRSA) invest in both fundamental training and emergency response public health workforce development. These programs evaluate training and education methods, provide evidence for the impact of training on capacity-building within public health agencies, and demonstrate methods for enhancing "competencies" in core public health practice, emergency preparedness, and other professional areas within the public health workforce. In addition to federal agency stakeholders, private associations have also promoted practice-based research. ASPH supports practice-based research between schools of public health and state and local public health departments through the funding of the ASPH Academic Health Departments (AHD). AHD are organized partnerships between schools of public health and health departments that create a dynamic academic/practice collaboration, which effectively pools assets of both institutions in the areas of teaching, research, and service. Academic/practice partnerships for research that use the AHD model can support the *reciprocal dynamic* process of teaching and learning by informing curricula and training through the new knowledge and practices gleaned from the outcomes of practice-based research.

Given the breadth of its scope and the diversity of its stakeholders, practice-based research has complex and inclusive conceptual foundations.

Four Elements of Research

Within any practice-based research paradigm, there are four elements that characterize how a systematic inquiry is pursued: approach, model, methods, and tools. All four elements are interactive, interlinked, and provide opportunities for feedback during the research endeavor. The graphic of the Four Elements of Research in Practice-Based Research illustrates the relationship between the four elements and is followed by discussion.

Research element: approach: As noted earlier, public health practice-based research uses multiple methodologies that may be qualitative and quantitative. The approach is the orientation of the investigator. For example, a hallmark approach of participatory research is its orientation to engage potential users, stakeholders, and beneficiaries in the research process. Another example of an approach in the basic or clinical research paradigms is hypothesis testing.

Research Element: Model

A model is the structured format and design that systematizes and operationalizes the research approach. Models help researchers explain, comprehend, discuss, organize, and manage complex public health problems in the natural world, in society, in individual behavior, or in organizations. According to Barbour, models are "neither literal pictures of reality nor 'useful fictions,' but partial and provisional ways of imagining what is not observable; they are symbolic representations of aspects of the world which are not directly accessible to us." In practice-based research, models are useful to help calculate disease and injury trends, determine population behaviours, and guide the development of interventions. For instance, if using a participatory research approach, one might select the community-based model that would engage the community in the research design. If using a systems research paradigm for agencies and organizations, one might use the Burke-Litwin model to plan and manage organizational change. If using a clinical paradigm, the model of clinical research teams from various disciplines, as exemplified at NIH, may be employed.

Demonstrating Excellence in Practice-based Research for Public Health

An important aspect of research models for public health practice is the extent to which they allow for collaboration among practitioners, community organizations, and academic researchers. Green and Mercer illustrate that models are affected by the degree of participation and types of research participant, and so will vary according to paradigm.

For example, defining the research question is the done by only the researchers in a basic research paradigm, but may involve multiple collaborators in a community research paradigm. The respective models for both basic and community research will therefore include standards of responsibility for problem definition within each paradigm.

Research element: methods: Methods are the structural guidelines used to implement the research model. A unique characteristic of practice-based research is consideration of the ecologic context of the research enterprise at some stage in the Cycle of the Practice-Based Research Process to ensure that the outcomes for the community are appropriate. Methods may be qualitative or quantitative in nature, as also seen in the research element "Approach," described earlier.

Using a Combination of Approaches and Methods to Solve Complex Public Health Problems

Real comprehension of public health problems and proposed solutions requires not only expert knowledge of the issue and its physical, social, cultural, and environmental impact on the involved populations, but also a comprehensive, multi-method research strategy to address the problem.

Morse discusses such a strategy called "methodological triangulation," which is the use of at least two methods (usually one that is qualitative and the other that is quantitative) to address the same research problem." Such a strategy allows the public health researchers (the academician and the practice partners are considered as co-equal researchers) the opportunity to apply scientific inquiry—induction, deduction, and verification—to address and resolve public health problems.

Research Element: Tools

Tools are the instruments or means used within a given research method. Tools measure the process and outcomes as linked to the research process.

The researcher can use tools innovatively for public health practice research. Many tools are available that are adaptable to practice-based research activities. On the qualitative side, there are case studies, key informant interviews, and client stories that document real life events in a narrative fashion and provide key data that can be used for the application of knowledge to inform the practice of care provision, service delivery, and policy development. On the quantitative side, the use of tools such as surveillance databases and public health opinion polls serve to both track the spread of disease and document the dissemination and effectiveness of health information.

Ethics Particular to Practice-based Research

All forms of research are constrained, focused, and balanced by ethical standards and methodological integrity. Practice-based research is no different, but it raises challenges for research ethics above and beyond those usual to most fields of science. Practice-based research supports or pursues at least seven of the twelve Principles of the Ethical Practice of Public Health. it addresses principally the fundamental causes of disease and requirements for health (Principle 1), respects the rights of individuals (Principle 2), ensures opportunities for input by community members (Principle 3), seeks information needed to implement effective policies and programs (Principle 5), provides communities with information (Principle 6), helps to ensure the professional competence of public health professionals (Principle 11), and engages public health institutions and their employees in collaborations that build the public's trust and the institution's effectiveness (Principle 12). Ethical standards for practice-based research may also be found in the "Ten Commandments for Community-based Research" and the four proposed ethical goals of community consultation by Dickert and Sugerman.

Research that engages those who are most concerned with and involved in public health problems has particularly serious challenges. For example, close collaboration with non-researchers increases the potential for disclosure and dissemination of information of a private or possibly detrimental nature for individuals and communities. Thus, practice-based research calls for rigorous compliance with state and federal privacy laws and institutional regulations.

Engagement of the community requires attention to the breadth and diversity of its values, beliefs, and cultures so that key partners and constituents are not unfairly overlooked or excluded. This necessitates efforts of relation-building and information-sharing that demand time and resources not necessarily essential to other kinds of research. Further, research results that point to ways of improving programs and policies impose an obligation on the researcher and the practitioner to implement those improvements for the benefit of community health and well-being. This suggests that practice-based research is ethically incomplete without attention to implementation and follow-through by researchers as well as non-researcher partners. As practice-based research is promoted and implemented, it is important to address the challenges of this research and its designs in receiving recognition and support as applied scholarship for academicians, as outlined in the 1999 ASPH Practice Council table "Challenges to Enabling Scholarly Practice in Schools of Public Health. In addition, offering quality incentives and expanded resources for practitioners and community partners will help address academic challenges and increase sustainability of academic/practice linkages for research.

The future of practice-based research rests on the capacity to develop and maintain stakeholder partnerships that are invested in its systems and institutions, in order to provide continuous funding and generate guidelines that sustain practice-based research. Practice-based research will thrive when it is institutionalized in research missions and guidelines within academic institutions so that rewards and benefits accrue to researchers, practitioners, and community participants. Incentives to create and refine methods and tools will assure the quality of the research and maintain rigor in solving new and emerging problems from the field. Attention to creating educational paths for students, researchers, and practitioners to attain competencies in practice-based research also helps expand this research. Finally, policies and strategies that facilitate the recognition and advancement of practice-based research, as well as reconcile the academic/practice tension, will also help sustain the practice-based research enterprise.

General Recommendations to Advance practice-based Research for Public Health

Provide Leadership Development in Practice-based Research

Leadership and advocacy will be required to advance the understanding, application, benefits and evaluation of practice-based research. Leadership strategies may include the following:

- o Develop and encourage interactive forums across disciplines, institutions, organizations, agencies, and the community to provide systematic opportunities for collaboration.
- o Develop and support institutional policies and practices, such as creating Memorandums of Understanding, that encourage practice-based research, recognize

organizational differences, and increase awareness of institutional review board (IRB) processes (e.g., in one ASPH Academic Health Department project, the school of public health developed guidelines on communication for practice-based research).

- o Collaborate with funders at all levels to assist in the dissemination of practice-based research to all stakeholders.

Enhance capacity building for practice-based research. The infrastructure for practice-based research includes building partnerships that are committed to the mutual benefit of the academy and community and supporting the evolution of researchers and practitioners. Capacity-building strategies may include the following:

- o Establish and enhance campus and community partnerships between academicians and practitioners for practice-based research.
- o Advocate for funding of practice-based research that recognizes the collaboration of agencies, organizations, foundations, and universities across diverse disciplines.
- o Build new research capacity through collaboration with newly identified community and university partners focused on community health problems.
- o Educate, recruit, provide leadership opportunities for, and reward practice-based researchers and practitioners through recognized career opportunities in health professions colleges, universities, and communities.

Medical Humanities

The field of MH developed in 1970s and included ethics, literature, history integrative medicine, and other topics, most often described from a physician's perspective. It was believed that, the approaches of medical humanities, particularly those drawn from philosophy and literature, would deepen and broaden understandings of healthcare. Thus the core subject of medicine would be supported by all other subjects on the periphery such as bioethics, religion, communication skills, theology, anthropology, forensic medicine, etc. and give new dimensions to medicine and medical practice. MH also includes many aspects relating to technological developments; for example test tube baby, surrogate motherhood, CT scan, PET scan etc.

A new focus on the importance of interdisciplinary education and collaborative experiences emerged enabling the medical fraternity to fully understand the patients, their diseases, sufferings and perceptions in relation to their culture, religious beliefs, values, feelings, fears and sufferings.

Communication skills are at the core the patient – physician relationship. In earlier days there was a strong bond between the family physician, the patient, and his family. He was involved in every family event and was well acquainted with the family issues related to health or other wise. Such practicing family physicians are now becoming rare probably due to the development, varied specializations, and the need for each individual to grow professionally and economically.

Specialized physicians are now, more involved in clinical research along with their routine of patient care. Much of clinical research is interdisciplinary in nature and is based on social aspects and follows social science research methodology such as, cohort studies, where collecting data without disturbing or hurting the individuals' psychology and feelings is of extreme importance.

MH in Literature

There are different views about MH in relation to medicine. One view is to regard medical ethics as one of the sub disciplines of medicine, while the other view believes that MH has a larger perspective. Medical Humanities educationists have argued that MH has two basic functions –a critical and analytical function and an educational function of enriching and developing the character. Ethical issues emerge from it as part of interdisciplinary approach to medical practice and theory. A third approach is to regard the medical humanities as a sustained exploration of both theory of knowledge (epistemology) and value-inquiry, as these are embodied in clinical medicine. Literature suggests that humanities might offer several benefits to clinicians. It would help by developing their abilities to communicate with patients, dwell deep in to their detailed narratives of illness, and eventually seek more diverse ways for patient's wellbeing and care. The recording and exploring human (patient) experiences, as in humanities, would help in better understanding of patient's illness, may help in treatment.

Cultural factors do influence people's health decision, and response to medical issues. Psychological social, spiritual and cultural taboos may differ with cultural variations and would need different approaches. Discussions on end of life or serious illness may be very challenging due to emotional and interpersonal intensity. For instance, decision on type of treatment in serious illness maybe taken by patient himself /herself, but in India the decision is often taken by the family members; or by spouse or jointly by the family, patient and the treating physician.

Although, whether patients demonstrably benefit from their practitioner's study of medical humanities is yet to be formally determined, there are strong theoretical reasons (as derived from literature) to believe that a practitioner with a broader understanding of medicine will be more effective.

Considering that all medical students should be humanists while practicing medicine, countries have felt it necessary to provide a broad based medical education. The aim of providing a broader medical education, covering humanities subjects, has been to produce kinder and more reflective practitioners. Medical Humanities teachers use literature while teaching medical students, to try to enliven discussion of medical ethics, discussion of religious issues, particularly surrounding bereavement. Ethics, health economics and medical anthropology have been considered by many schools as important peripheral subjects of medicine.

A series of articles on end of life and religious beliefs in Lancet 2005 is a testimony of the need of knowledge about MH in medicine. These articles focused on the end of life and issues of bereaved family members, and the religious beliefs of several faiths. The authors have suggested that if the care taker is knowledgeable about these beliefs, taking care of patients and supporting the family members is much easier, and acceptable. It is observed that serious illness or in cases of imminent death, patient and family members pursue spiritual ways to come to terms with life and near death situations. Similarly, the December issue of Indian journal of Palliative care published two articles on end of life and spiritual perspectives.

Both the articles emphasize the challenging issues surrounding the end of life care especially related to psychological, social and cultural dimensions. They suggest that palliative care practitioners must be sensitive to and have appreciation of different religious perspectives and rituals to meet unique needs of their patients and families. There are world wide variations in the perspectives on life, suffering, death, and after life. It is therefore suggested that better understanding of the traditions, common rituals surrounding the death and rebirth, ritual after death, and bereavement can improve care for patients and their family members. This avoids practitioners from imposing their convictions and faith and be proactive in their spiritual needs and help patient in achieving 'good death' and at the same time help family members to deal with the grief. Providing a culture sensitive care is extremely essential. Cultural variations, values and attitudes have important practical implications for individuals responsible for making critical medical decisions. Articles on holistic approach for elderly care in Indian situations ; an overview on Palliative care / home care on beliefs and end of life , on spirituality and end of life and many other articles, all point towards the need to understand these issues for better and satisfactory care of patients.

There are other situations such as 'labeling patients' or 'labeling persons' either during care or when diagnosing. Each patient has different perceptions related to his/ her health. Keeping this in mind, the care taker should carefully handle the 'labeling' of patient, as it can cause a long term psychological impact. Understanding human behavior and the different human personalities should help medical practitioners in handling situations with care and positive impact.

This concept is not limited to individual health care personnel or clinicians, but is extended to organizations as well. Literature has indicated that organizational systems have to be sensitive to cultural diversity and variations and also should have linguistic competency, to be able meet patient's cultural, social and communication needs.

MH knowledge is applicable, to address effectively, the disclosure of bad news, informed consent, confidentiality, dishonesty, research ethics, end-of-life care, resource allocation and the like. The doctor must recognize situations as an ethical dilemma; possess the relevant knowledge of cultural norms, laws and policies; analyze how this knowledge applies to the situation at hand; and demonstrate the skills needed to communicate and negotiate this situation in practice.

It is well known fact that most of diseases are locality and region oriented. The health care centres situated in these areas are aware of the regional features, local people, their cultures, religions and customs, are prepared with required kits (diagnostic and treatment drugs) and health care programme are designed, depending upon the community it serves. The knowledge of MH would also help in education, application and promotion on issues with social impact like cryopreservation.

Relevance of MH in India

India is a diverse country in terms of religion and faith, culture, languages, beliefs, life styles, eating habits, rituals, superstitions, economic status, etc. It is sometimes found that this diversity has resulted in an integration of traditions between cultures. It is expected of clinicians to be aware of cultural diversity and beliefs and to provide culturally sensitive care especially in end-of life care practices. In cancer hospitals, palliative and / or end of life care is offered as an integral part of patient care. To support such information needs, which presently are not clearly defined, but are taking shape indirectly through efforts of Institutional Review Board (IRB) activities, Non Governmental Organizations (NGOs), patient and consumer education, and consumer courts, the hospital libraries have to be well equipped with collections in MH.

In recent years, India is becoming a centre for clinical medical tourism. Clinical research, usually sponsored by pharma industry is also rapidly increasing and the country is now flooded with clinical studies both drug trials and other forms of clinical research. With the large patient base, various diseases, improving infrastructure, industry friendly regulations, strong ethical guidelines and trained workforce, India has become a centre for clinical trials for many international companies and the growth is only likely to increase in future. However, to achieve its goal of becoming a global hub of clinical trials, the country will have to overcome challenges like unethical trials.

The world's top ten global pharma industries are currently carrying out the largest number of clinical trials in India. It has been reported that of total trials registered in US, 8.9% are conducted in Asia, 7.4 % Latin Am., 7.1 % Central and Eastern Europe and 1.6% in Africa. If only India is to be considered, it is observed that the major players are GSK (122), U K based industry, Astra Zeneca (186), Johnson and Johnson, Pfizer, and many more from companies like – Wyeth, Merck, Bristol-Myers, etc. covering drugs and vaccine trials including patients and participants from all age groups and often include women of childbearing age. It is estimated that by 2011 India will be conducting more than 15% of trials conducted globally.

Clinical trials definitely have an advantage for outsourced developing countries. They bring in new technology and new treatments and they also sensitize the biomedical community towards the country's need to advance medical and clinical research. Several times established drugs are studied .The whole process is viewed in Indian settings, in terms of safety of people, economics, culture, and need, to satisfy the regulatory requirements of the land (Drug Controller General of India).

The study medications are often offered free to patients / participants, who might benefit from such drugs. So there is an advantage to the patients and the community as well.

There is a well developed and established Ethical Guidelines to be followed in order to ensure safety of participants; it is essential that, people who conduct trials, design trials and who administer consent and also those who review the projects for ethical approval are knowledgeable about various ethical issues. India is now facing the challenges of protecting trial participants and patient care, keeping in view the differences in cultural and spiritual outlooks to life.

While there was no registry of clinical trials and people were really not aware of how many similar studies were being conducted and by whom. Recently, the Government of India (ICMR) initiated the registration of all clinical studies including PG student research, which have to be evaluated for scientific and ethical issues. Bioethics does not simply relate to protecting participants' health – psychological, and physical; but its objective is to protect all aspects of the participants – physical, psychological, economical, religious beliefs, faith and cultural, as well. This calls for researchers who can understand these aspects. Clinicians or researchers are required to have information and knowledge not only about participants' safety but also about their socio-cultural backgrounds and beliefs. It is essential that the researcher respects the human side of medicine and research. The participants should also be well aware about the studies, their rights and responsibilities, risks and benefits that may come to them.

The need for medical professionals to understand this 'humane' aspect of patients has been long established and many of western medical / health science institutes have included Medical Humanities (MH) in their curricula. However, in India MH has not entered the medical curriculum either at the undergraduate or post graduate stage.

The fact that publications related to spirituality and patient care have appeared in national scholarly / scientific publications are indications that India too is recognizing the need of medical humanities and organizations should encourage and allow the libraries to support such activities through its collection and services. Libraries should support these activities and needs of newer directives of the national polices, through collection. But, presently the libraries are neither encouraged to collect such broad based resources nor do their budgets allow them to support collection of materials other than the main domain of the hospital requirements. With these developments in medical practice and research, it is essential that collection development policy of a hospital library should be redefined to incorporate the collection of humanities. Queries on various aspects of MH were put to the author and the information could only be provided with help from Social science research libraries within the city. These experiences triggered interest in the field. In a cancer hospital, healing is often supported by the benefits of collaborative medicine and its enhancement through art therapy, e.g. - music therapy. It emphasizes meeting the psychosocial needs of patients, encouraging participation in treatment, and facilitating a psychologically positive hospital experience through the application of music, exchange of thoughts of patient groups, etc. It has been observed by many that psychological symptoms, such as depression and anxiety, commonly experienced by patients with chronic illness, are satisfactorily dealt through the creative arts programs. The specific physical and psychological benefits of music, in oncology treatment have been recorded in medical literature. The rehabilitation centre / unit of most of the hospitals indulge in several such activities with patients, particularly with children. It promotes drawing, paintings and even musical events, where the patients are participants. These are actually a form of therapy and give an additive effect for the response to medical treatment. These forms of activities are gaining ground in hospitals in India and when such activities are undertaken and promoted by the organization, it is necessary that the library supports the need by providing books and such other materials.

Clinical studies are often related to social aspects, results of which may affect public health policies. e.g., behavioural studies of patients, public health surveys, etc. Several such studies are based on social science methodology and evaluated based on standard keys. e.g., perceptions of pain, scale to evaluate sexual function after treatment of gynecologic cancer, etc.

A Review

With these issues and needs in view, a study of the collection development policy of major hospitals, medical college and research centre libraries in the city of Mumbai was undertaken. Libraries of ten major hospitals (which were also teaching institutes) in the city were selected,, on the basis of their budgets and total collection, for the survey. A small questionnaire was served to the library chiefs. Of the ten major libraries, two institutes were a century old, seven had completed about 50-70 years of establishment and the remaining one was less than a decade old. In all cases the libraries were established since the inception of the institutes. The questionnaire related to the present collection and the collection development policy, (particularly in relation to collection of medical humanities). The participants were provided with a brief about the study, its purpose and possible outcomes. Following observations were made –

1. There were four under graduate teaching institutes while the remaining were post graduate institutes, MH was not included in the curricula, at either level. But two teaching institutes conducted workshops for junior doctors on 'how to communicate with patients. These workshops covered some aspects of MH, particularly how to ask questions for better understanding of their illness. At these workshops librarians participated.

2. All the institutes had an institutional review board (IRB), a rehabilitation centre and medical social workers to assist patients. All the institutes were engaged in clinical research – funded in-house or extramural funds or were supported by pharma companies. This showed that there was definitely a need for MH information; but hospital libraries were not approached. In any case they did not have any resources to meet these needs.

3. It was found that except for one, none of the libraries had a well defined written collection development policy. However each one of them were following some unwritten criteria and guidelines, which had developed out of situations; the suggestions and recommendations of the library committees were generally accepted. Few of the major points were -

   a. It was the practice in most libraries to equally distribute the budget amongst the departments in the hospital. This was an arrangement to make the selection and purchase a balanced one and, to some extent, to satisfy the needs of different users. However the budget always needed to be redistributed / adjusted during the year to accommodate the purchase of a series or reference volumes such as encyclopedias; the cost of these was met by drawing funds from the unused allocations of different departments.

b. The recommending authorities were usually the department or unit heads, however the final decision lay with the library committee and the head of the institute. The libraries did not cover MH subjects, although there were departments such as preventive medicine, IRB, rehabilitation, social work, etc.,

c. The library collections focused on all aspects of medical specialties, and criteria for selection for almost all libraries were similar, –

   i. Text books as required by and prescribed for undergraduates and post graduates, only latest edition were acquired.

   ii. Advanced research books and journals as required by faculties, depending upon their research activities.

   iii. Journals (both print and electronic) were subscribed covering all specialties and continuity in subscriptions was maintained as permissible by budget. The subscriptions were usually print plus electronic based.

   iv. Few libraries had initiated joint subscriptions to some commonly subscribed journals.

4. Almost all librarians received requests for information other than medicine, mainly on general management, engineering, human behavior, forensic law, and ethical issues. The library collection did not support such queries and the librarians had felt the need of developing MH collection.

5. The libraries, except for one, did not specifically make any attempt to add subjects related to arts and humanities but had a small collection related to forensic law, since this was usually a part of the curriculum. The single library

which collected a few books on MH was fairly new. In the past two years it had collected less than 150 books but no journals on MH. No new additions were being made.

6. Two major libraries reported that during the initial years the library did collect some books and a few journal titles in the areas of social and behavioural sciences. During the early 1990s, the additions and subscriptions to these were discontinued due to budget constraints. Of late due to rise in clinical research and the mandate of IRB approval, the need to develop a collection on MH was deeply felt and expressed by the library committee. However, in practice, the collection had not been developed for want of additional budget. The libraries yet maintain small collections of 'holistic medicine' under which donated items on such subjects are classified.

7. Library professionals suggested that following aspects should be addressed in the guidelines for collection of MH:
   a. Special budget allocations be made for books, journals, e- resources etc.
   b. Identification of recommending authority, since the subject would be of relevance to all
   c. Coverage or scope of collection
   d. Structure on how to conceptualize and develop such a collection.

Collection development of Medical Humanities has to be done objectively, since the subject would relate to all aspects of patient care and research, from local and community information to communication skills, religious beliefs and faith to ethical issues. A policy on collection development of peripheral nature of the subject needs a careful attention. The policy should aim at avoiding over enthusiasm or should not be event driven. It should be framed to support organization activity and user needs. According to the guidelines of IFLA, a policy should clearly define the audience for whom the collection is being developed, purpose of such collection, description of collection, levels or depths and limitations of collection and local importance.

Guidelines for Policy Development

The mandate of any medical / health science library is to concentrate on medical collection covering all specialties. There are several issues to be addressed while developing a policy to cover the inclusion of MH in the collection. The following points/ questions may need to be answered in order to formulate the policy. These would need to be further fine tuned, depending upon the community the hospital serves, the hospital activities and needs and the queries that are made on the library.

Specify the Target Group

The core group of users would obviously be the clinical faculty of the institution. In addition, should the library, cater to the needs of non-clinical staff, external consultants, patients and their families, NGOs working with patients, public health departments, and such others?

Decide on the Scope

Should all humanities subjects, which have implications for the medical profession be acquired? Specific decisions on the following areas may need to be taken - anthropology, behavioural sciences, bioethics; medical law; social issues, health economics; spirituality, religion; literature like short stories of life experiences, fictions and books with specific purposes for example "chicken soup for the soul" series may need to be taken, Books on happiness and religious customs, culture and lifestyle may also be considered. Within these broad areas, focus should be on the specific communities of the neighborhood.

HR Management in Hospitals: An Overview

Handling Human Resources in Hospitals

Human resource plays a very significant role in effective performance of a hospital which depends to a great extent on the quality of its staff. The better the quality, the higher the level of performance. Hospital is a place where, on one hand, we have highly skilled personnel such as doctors and on the other, we have unskilled workers such as sweepers. Management has been using the traditional tools which are basically coercive in nature (such as, punishment, suspension, degradation and discharge) to control the employees but it is to be realised that these coercive measures are never productive.

To control the staff effectively, modern management tools are to be adopted and coercive measures are to be replaced by persuasive ones. Let me illustrate it by an example. Suppose, a sweeper in a hospital is not in the habit of cleaning the lavatory on daily basis. He does it when told/reminded to do so. If you remind him everyday, he will clean it everyday. If you do not tell, he does not do. How are you going to tackle this problem? Those who believe in old management theory will follow the course of action as follow herewith: a) call the sweeper, b) describe him the problem, c) warn him of punishment if he does not perform/ improve, and d) take action which may include removal from the job, if he does not show improvement. On the other hand, the management which practices the principle of persuasion will tackle the problem in a different way. They will talk to the sweeper, let him feel how important his job is and hence how important he is for the hospital. Such an approach will have a lasting impact on his mind.

If necessary, short class room lectures may be held where the matters such as nosocomial infections etc. may be discussed. Having done so, a close watch may be kept on him. If necessary, one person may be deployed who will be after him to make sure that he cleans the toilet everyday. In all likelihood, he will improve and cleaning toilets on everyday basis will become his habit. So, the focus should be on converting the duties of staff into their habits. Once the habits are formed, there is no need for reminders/ supervision and the staff will become a very valuable asset for the hospital.

Management also faces problems in dealing with doctors. There will be a different set of problems while handling them. Doctors, to some extent, may like to be controlled by a senior doctor manager but not by a non-doctor manager.

There are many reasons for the same and they need to be analysed before any line of action is chalked out. Doctors perhaps have education/knowledge superiority when compared with management professionals. They do not consider the management professionals at par with them and therefore, there is a problem of adjustment. From the begining, the subject 'healthcare' has been under the control of state/central government. Public hospitals have doctors designated as medical superintendent who take care of the day to day administration of the hospitals. So, doctors have been playing dual role. Now, it has been felt that healthcare institutions are not delivering results largely due to inefficient management.

Therefore there is a trend to bring management professionals for hospital administration/management jobs. Doctors may not have much say in routine administrative matters and therefore, they are resisting the changes although they, too, are very much convinced that they are not best suited for management jobs and it will be in overall interest if they concentrate on clinical jobs only. Not being in the management job may lessen their authority/ power on hospital staff and they find it difficult to accept these changes. Doctors are not taught management in medical colleges. For them, hospital means doctor and doctor means hospital. So, they are not educationally equipped to appreciate the roles of management professionals in hospital administration. 4) Doctors were respected in the society. Now, monetary and other related factors have eroded this position. There is customer-supplier relationship between the patient and the doctor. Service of a doctor has become a commodity which is being sold off.

Therefore, a need is being felt to hand over the management jobs to management experts only. Doctors, now, have started realising it. So, doctors and management both need to change their attitude towards each other. Also, the management professionals need to introduce the essence of participative management while dealing with doctors. Doctors simply must not be ignored on the ground that it is none of their business. CME programme of doctors, too, need to be modified. Apart from the clinical subjects, CME should cover the various areas of hospital management. They should also cover the subjects such as 'development of personality traits' and similar other topics so that it can prepare the doctors to adapt themselves easily to the need of hours.

Also, there is need to develop positive attitude towards all the jobs of the hospital. A doctor may have to be in operation theatre, say foı six hours and it may at appear tough but there is no shortcut to it. Similarly, a hospital administrator sits in the office and manages the affairs from there. There must not be seen any luxury in it. It is the demand of management profession. He can not move now and then. He has to sit in the office and keep watch on various activities going on in the hospital. Since, he is virtually responsible for everything in the hospital, he can not assign all the tasks to himself. He has to delegate and keep the control in his hands and play the role of a co-ordinator. Now, no comparison should be made between two jobs. The underlining spirit should be - all jobs are important. Therefore, handling the staff is a real challenging job.

Sacking/suspension/discharge is a easy way out to get rid of the staff we do not like but retaining them in job is a real difficult job and only an able hospital administrator can do it.

Strategies for Assisting Health Workers to Modify and Improve Akills: Developing Quality Health Care - A Process of Change

Health care workers all over the world are facing difficult challenges. The public's expectation of them continues to rise. Yet as a result of fiscal constraints, often created by worsening economic conditions, they are asked to provide more, higher quality health services with fewer resources. At the same time, the knowledge and skills-base needed to perform effectively in their chosen fields of endeavour continues to grow and change rapidly. Health care personnel will continue in the workforce for many years, while the information that they acquired during their education may rapidly become obsolete.

Health care institutions and their managers are also confronted with these realities. The challenge is to continue to maintain or improve the quality of the care provided and maintain, or even expand, the comprehensiveness of health service coverage, while introducing changes in care delivery or service mix necessitated by reduced budgets.

Finally, governments at local, regional and national levels are attempting to obtain greater value for the money they spend on health care. Faced with growing expectations of quality, they are being asked to be more accountable for the results of their health care expenditures. Thus, they also have an important role to play in ensuring and improving the quality of health services provided in both the public and private sectors.

What is Quality Health Care?

There are many different definitions of quality in health care. The characteristics emphasized vary according to the perspectives of the different stakeholders involved in crafting the definition and in determining how the definition is to be used.

Definitions of quality of care include such characteristics as efficiency, efficacy, effectiveness, equity, accessibility, comprehensiveness, acceptability, timeliness, appropriateness, continuity, privacy and confidentiality.

Other attributes that have been used to describe quality health care include provisions of education for the patient and family about pertinent health issues, inclusion of the patient and family in treatment planning and decision-making, and patient satisfaction. Ensuring safety and support in the care environment, reducing mortality and morbidity and improving the quality of life and functional health status of the patient may also be seen as quality attributes.

Achieving Quality:Building or Inspecting it?

Two different approaches have been taken in monitoring the quality of care with the aim of improving it: quality assurance and quality improvement. Although both rely on performance monitoring, they differ in how indicators of quality are selected, the emphasis that they place on having criteria or standards by which to gauge aspects of the structure, process or outcomes of care, and the way the information obtained is used.

Quality assurance (QA), the older of the approaches, emphasizes meeting or exceeding agreed upon minimum standards of performance which are usually set by an individual or group external to those who are to be assessed. The criteria it uses may be implicit or explicit. When explicit criteria for performance are set, these are usually based on the best available scientific and clinical evidence.

Agreement of experts may also be used to set criteria but serious questions have been raised about the validity of this approach because their consensus does not always coincide with the best available medical evidence. This approach is useful when the evidence is conflicting, ambiguous or lacking.

The aim of quality assurance is to make certain that the criteria set are being met. Thus, action on the part of the health professional (to improve performance to reach the level of the standard or criterion) is only demanded when the facility, service or person whose performance is assessed does not meet the minimal standard.

Sometimes, failure to meet the standard results in reprimands, close monitoring, fines or other sanctions such as temporary loss of licence to carry out such activities. Usually, some remedial action plan is developed that is agreed upon by the parties and performance is reassessed after a given time period. Because QA emphasizes finding and correcting problems, it can be perceived as a negatively-oriented process. Many health care professionals are unenthusiastic about it as they perceive it as a threat to, rather than as a support for, their work activities.

Quality improvement (QI) represents a paradigm shift away from a major concern with inspection of activities and detection of those care providers (clinics, health care teams, hospitals, etc.) who fail to meet minimal criteria or standards to an emphasis on continuous positive change in performance.

The underlying philosophy of QI is that no matter how good care is, it can always be improved. QI assumes that health care providers are concerned about doing a good job and want to do the best job possible. Processes, particularly interfaces between different aspects of the process of care, are often problematic and, when these are identified, solutions can be found to make care more effective, efficient, humane, and geared to the preferences of patients and their families.

Factors that Influence Quality of Care

The way the health care system is structured, including the number and types of health care personnel available, and how they are deployed and distributed, can all influence the quality of the services delivered.

The pace at which change is occurring, the availability of technology needed to deliver quality care, and the expertise and style of health care resource management available may also influence quality. Entry-level knowledge, skills and understandings of health care workers are affected by the quality of the basic educational system, the links between the health education and health care sectors and the extent to which the educational system promotes continuing learning skills and models multi-disciplinary cooperation. The ability of the existing workforce to acquire new skills may also be limited by the support available through the educational system (e.g. library, courses, distance learning opportunities).

Tools to help Health Care Personnel Improve Quality

A wide variety of strategies are used in quality assurance or improvement. Some target health care personnel directly while others affect the quality of care delivered by providers more indirectly. Such strategies may target the structure or process of the health care or health education system, either at the local level or at regional/national level, and thus have indirect effects on health care personnel.

Tools that target providers directly include unsolicited mailings of information, academic detailing of new information, use of educational influence, hospital "rounds", development of standards of practice, practice guidelines and care-maps, reminder systems built into practice records, computer-based interventions, or peer audit and feedback based on guidelines, and a plethora of other types of formal and informal continuing education opportunities.

Self- and peer-assessment of learning needs are often used to help the learner determine what learning needs should be addressed.

At the local health care delivery level, numerous activities may be used in an effort to enhance quality. They include adopting standards, guidelines and care-maps, forming standing committees to monitor key work activities and giving credentials to professional employees.

Quality improvement initiatives may involve job/process re-engineering or cross-training of workers. Management and clinical information systems may be developed. Workers may be given leave to attend continuing education courses. Establishment of criteria for renewal of licence or job appointments may also induce health care personnel to review knowledge/skill needs and increase the likelihood that they will seek ways of continuing their own learning.

At the regional or national level, policies and legislation regarding the health care delivery system or the educational system for health personnel, including continuing education, may be devised to improve quality. New or changed legislation that governs the education of health care personnel, the mandate and operations of the health care system and its institutions, and the scope of practice and regulation of the various health professions can have far-reaching effects on quality of care, including improving the quality of health professionals' knowledge, skills and activities.

However, these effects are not likely to be accomplished by such strategies alone. Legislation provides a framework within which change can be promoted and managed. Health care workers should also have access to the tools and resources needed to increase their knowledge and change their behaviour.

The Importance of Environmental Factors

Provider behaviour is influenced by the immediate environment (e.g. private office, group practice or public facility) and interaction with the patients, staff and co-workers in that environment.

Enabling and reinforcing features can be built into this environment as described later in section 4. It is more difficult to influence the personal environment of a practitioner, but we must be aware that this also influences behaviour. The educational environment consists of the way the educational system is structured with regard to basic, advanced and continuing education. This environment helps to shape the kinds of learning opportunities that are provided.

The professional environment consists of professional colleagues and associations (including certifying, credentialing and licensing bodies). The professional environment often alerts the provider to new and important developments in the field of practice and tries to promote the profession.

It may also assist the provider in changing behaviour by sponsoring continuing education activities. Regulatory bodies may offer incentives and place limits with sanctions on provider behaviour. The community environment determines how practitioners are perceived in the wider community; the media, local decision-makers responsible for health and health care, and opinion leaders help shape this environment.

The administrative environment determines the kinds of rules and regulations that govern aspects such as practitioner behaviour, working conditions, health education and health care facilities. It creates a broad set of incentives and sanctions for providers and makes them accountable for their actions. The administrative environment can be divided into local, regional and national levels, and is created by structures and processes at each of these levels. They are ultimately informed and influenced by the broader culture and by specific policies and legislation. Finally, as the broader social, cultural, economic and political environment is likely to have an indirect influence, only policies and legislation directly related to health care personnel will be considered.

Healthcare in India

Healthcare in India is the responsibility of constituent states and territories of India. The Constitution charges every state with "raising of the level of nutrition and the standard of living of its people and the improvement of public health as among its primary duties". The National Health Policy was endorsed by the Parliament of India in 1983 and updated in 2002.

The art of Health Care in India can be traced back nearly 3500 years. From the early days of Indian history the Aryurvedic tradition of medicine has been practiced. During the rule of Emperor Ashoka Maurya (third century B.C.E.), schools of learning in the healing arts were created. Many valuable herbs and medicinal combinations were created. Even today many of these continue to be used. During his rein there is evidence that Emperor Ashoka was the first leader in world history to attempt to give health care to all of his citizens, thus it was the India of antiquity which was the first state to give it's citizens national health care.

In recent times India has eradicated mass famines, half of children in India are underweight, one of the highest rates in the world and nearly the same rate of Sub-Saharan Africa.

Water supply and sanitation in India continue to be a challenge, only one of three Indians has access to improved sanitation facilities such as toilet. India's HIV/AIDS epidemic is a growing threat. Cholera epidemics are not unknown. The maternal mortality in India is the second highest in the world.

Providing healthcare and disease prevention to India's growing population of more than a billion people becomes challenging in the face of increased competition for resources. 2.47 million people in India are estimated to be HIV positive.

India is one of the four countries worldwide where polio has not as yet been successfully eradicated and one third of the world's tuberculosis cases are in India. Three out of four children who died from measles in 2008 were in India. According to the World Health Organization 900,000 Indians die each year from drinking contaminated water and breathing in polluted air. As India grapples with these basic issues, new challenges are emerging for example there is a rise in chronic adult diseases such as cardiovascular illnesses and diabetes as a consequence of changing lifestyles.

There are vast disparities in people's health even among the different states across the country largely attributed to the resource allocation by the state governments where some states have been more successful than others. Critics say better efforts are needed by the local governments to ensure that the health services provided are actually reaching the poor in worst-affected areas.

However, at the same time, India's health care system also includes entities which are world class. India is a magnet for medical tourists, who are able to get medical treatments and surgeries at a fraction of the cost of these procedures in developed countries.

The Apollo set of hospitals, for example, thrives on this business. Each hospital, however, must also set aside a number of beds for the poor. However, as the BBC reported, access to these services by the poor is plagued with corruption. While many foreign medical experts criticize medical tourism, many private hospitals are able to demonstrate that their level of care is comparable, if not better, than that received in developed countries.

Medical Professionals

In a 2005 World Bank study, World Bank reported that "a detailed survey of the knowledge of medical practitioners for treating five common conditions in Delhi found that the average doctor in a public primary health centre has around a 50-50 chance of recommending a harmful treatment". Random visits by government inspectors showed that 40% of public sector medical workers were not found at the workplace.

Neurosurgery

Modern neurosurgery in India begins in 1949, with the return of Jacob Chandy to the Christian Medical College, Vellore. Stereotactic surgery for pain, epilepsy, behaviour disorders and involuntary movements is being practised at several centres especially at Madras. As of 1983, there were about 180 neurosurgeons in India, or one for 3.6 million people.

Diseases

Ongoing government of India education about HIV has led to decreases in the spread of HIV in recent years. The number of people living with AIDS in India is estimated to be between 2 and

3 million. However in terms of the total population this is a small number. The country has had a sharp decrease in the estimated number of HIV infections; 2005 reports had claimed that there were 5.2 million to 5.7 million people afflicted with the virus.

Malnutrition

Half of children in India are underweight, one of the highest rates in the world and nearly same as Sub-Saharan Africa. India contributes to about 5.6 million child deaths every year, more than half the world's total.

Women

Most Indian women are malnourished. The average female life expectancy today in India is low compared to many countries, but it has shown gradual improvement over the years. In many families, especially rural ones, the girls and women face nutritional discrimination within the family, and are anemic and malnourished.

The maternal mortality in India is the second highest in the world. Only 42% of births in the country are supervised by health professionals. Most women deliver with help from women in the family who often lack the skills and resources to save the mother's life if it is in danger. According to UNDP Human Development Report (1997), 88% of pregnant women (age 15-49) were found to be suffering from anemia.

Water and Sanitation

Water supply and sanitation in India continue to be abysmal, despite longstanding efforts by the various levels of government and communities at improving coverage. The situation is particularly inadequate for sanitation, since only one of three Indians has access to improved sanitation facilities (including improved latrines).

While the share of those with access to an improved water source is much higher than for sanitation (86%), the quality of service is poor and most users that are counted as having access receive water of dubious quality and only on an intermittent basis. As of 2003, it was estimated that only 30% of India's wastewater was being treated, with the remainder flowing into rivers or groundwater. The lack of toilet facilities in many areas also presents a major health risk; open defecation is widespread even in urban areas of India, and it was estimated in 2002 by the World Health Organisation that around 700,000 Indians die each year from diarrhoea. No city in India has full-day water supply. Most cities supply water only a few hours a day. In towns and rural areas the situation is even worse.

Healthcare Infrastructure

The Indian healthcare industry is seen to be growing at a rapid pace and is expected to become a Us." billion industry by 2022. The Indian healthcare market was estimated at US$35 billion in 2007 and is expected to reach over US$70 billion by 2012 and Us." billion by 2017.

According to the Investment Commission of India the healthcare sector has experienced phenomenal growth of 12 percent per annum in the last 4 years. Rising income levels and a growing elderly population are all factors that are driving this growth. In addition, changing demographics, disease profiles and the shift from chronic to lifestyle diseases in the country has led to increased spending on healthcare delivery.

Even so, the vast majority of the country suffers from a poor standard of healthcare infrastructure which has not kept up with the growing economy. Despite having centres of excellence in healthcare delivery, these facilities are limited and are inadequate in meeting the current healthcare demands. Most public health facilities lack efficiency, are understaffed and have poorly maintained or outdated medical equipment.

Approximately one million people, mostly women and children, die in India each year due to inadequate healthcare. 700 million people have no access to specialist care and 80% of specialists live in urban areas. In addition to poor infrastructure India faces a shortage of trained medical personal especially in rural areas where access to care is altogether limited.

In order to meet manpower shortages and reach world standards India would require investments of up to $20 billion over the next 5 years. Forty percent of the primary health centres in India are understaffed. According to WHO statistics there are over 250 medical colleges in the modern system of medicine and over 400 in the Indian system of medicine and homeopathy (ISM&H).

India produces over 250,000 doctors annually in the modern system of medicine and a similar number of ISM&H practitioners, nurses and para professionals. Better policy regulations and the establishment of public private partnerships are possible solutions to the problem of manpower shortage.

India faces a huge need gap in terms of availability of number of hospital beds per 1000 population. With a world average of 3.96 hospital beds per 1000 population India stands just a little over 0.7 hospital beds per 1000 population.

Moreover, India faces a shortage of doctors, nurses and paramedics that are needed to propel the growing healthcare industry. India is now looking at establishing academic medical centres (AMCs) for the delivery of higher quality care with leading examples of The Manipal Group & All India Institute of Medical Sciences (AIIMS) already in place.

As incomes rise and the number of available financing options in terms of health insurance policies increase, consumers become more and more engaged in making informed decisions about their health and are well aware of the costs associated with those decisions. In order to remain competitive, healthcare providers are now not only looking at improving operational efficiency but are also looking at ways of enhancing patient experience overall.

Central Government Role

Critics say that the national policy lacks specific measures to achieve broad stated goals. Particular problems include the failure to integrate health services with wider economic and social development, the lack of nutritional support and sanitation, and the poor participatory involvement at the local level.

Central government efforts at influencing public health have focused on the five-year plans, on coordinated planning with the states, and on sponsoring major health programs. Government expenditures are jointly shared by the central and state governments.

Goals and strategies are set through central-state government consultations of the Central Council of Health and Family Welfare. Central government efforts are administered by the Ministry of Health and Family Welfare, which provides both administrative and technical services and manages medical education. States provide public services and health education.

The 1983 National Health Policy is committed to providing health services to all by 2000. In 1983 health care expenditures varied greatly among the states and union territories, from Rs. 13 per capita in Bihar to Rs. 60 per capita in Himachal Pradesh, and Indian per capita expenditure was low when compared with other Asian countries outside of South Asia.

Although government health care spending progressively grew throughout the 1980s, such spending as a percentage of the gross national product (GNP) remained fairly constant. In the meantime, health care spending as a share of total government spending decreased. During the same period, private-sector spending on health care was about 1.5 times as much as government spending.

Expenditure

In the mid-1990s, health spending amounted to 6% of GDP, one of the highest levels among developing nations. The established per capita spending is around Rs. 320 per year with the major input from private households (75%).

State governments contribute 15.2%, the central government 5.2%, third-party insurance and employers 3.3%, and municipal government and foreign donors about 1.3, according to a 1995 World Bank study. Of these proportions, 58.7% goes toward primary health care (curative, preventive, and promotive) and 38.8% is spent on secondary and tertiary inpatient care. The rest goes for nonservice costs.

The fifth and sixth five-year plans (FY 1974-78 and FY 1980-84, respectively) included programs to assist delivery of preventive medicine and improve the health status of the rural population. Supplemental nutrition programs and increasing the supply of safe drinking water were high priorities. The sixth plan aimed at training more community health workers and increasing efforts to control communicable diseases. There were also efforts to improve regional imbalances in the distribution of health care resources.

The Seventh Five-Year Plan (FY 1985-89) budgeted Rs. 33.9 billion for health, an amount roughly double the outlay of the sixth plan. Health spending as a portion of total plan outlays, however, had declined over the years since the first plan in 1951, from a high of 3.3% of the total plan spending in FY 1951-55 to 1.9% of the total for the seventh plan. Mid-way through the Eighth Five-Year Plan (FY 1992-96), however, health and family welfare was budgeted at Rs. 20 billion, or 4.3% of the total plan spending for FY 1994, with an additional Rs. 3.6 billion in the nonplan budget.

Primary Services

Health care facilities and personnel increased substantially between the early 1950s and early 1980s, but because of fast population growth, the number of licensed medical practitioners per 10,000 individuals had fallen by the late 1980s to three per 10,000 from the 1981 level of four per 10,000. In 1991 there were approximately ten hospital beds per 10,000 individuals. However for comparison, the in China for comparison there are 1.4 doctors per 1000 people.

Primary health centres are the cornerstone of the rural health care system. By 1991, India had about 22,400 primary health centres, 11,200 hospitals, and 27,400 clinics. These facilities are part of a tiered health care system that funnels more difficult cases into urban hospitals while attempting to provide routine medical care to the vast majority in the countryside.

Primary health centres and subcenters rely on trained paramedics to meet most of their needs. The main problems affecting the success of primary health centres are the predominance of clinical and curative concerns over the intended emphasis on preventive work and the reluctance of staff to work in rural areas. In addition, the integration of health services with family planning programs often causes the local population to perceive the primary health centres as hostile to their traditional preference for large families. Therefore, primary health centres often play an adversarial role in local efforts to implement national health policies.

According to data provided in 1989 by the Ministry of Health and Family Welfare, the total number of civilian hospitals for all states and union territories combined was 10,157. In 1991 there was a total of 811,000 hospital and health care facilities beds. The geographical distribution of hospitals varied according to local socio-economic conditions. In India's most populous state, Uttar Pradesh, with a 1991 population of more than 139 million, there were 735 hospitals as of 1990. In Kerala, with a 1991 population of 29 million occupying an area only one-seventh the size of Uttar Pradesh, there were 2,053 hospitals.

Although central government has set a goal of health care for all by 2000, hospitals are distributed unevenly. Private studies of India's total number of hospitals in the early 1990s were more conservative than official Indian data, estimating that in 1992 there were 7,300 hospitals.

Of this total, nearly 4,000 were owned and managed by central, state, or local governments. Another 2,000, owned and managed by charitable trusts, received partial support from the government, and the remaining 1,300 hospitals, many of which were relatively small facilities, were owned and managed by the private sector. The use of state-of-the-art medical equipment, often imported from Western countries, was primarily limited to urban centres in the early 1990s.

A network of regional cancer diagnostic and treatment facilities was being established in the early 1990s in major hospitals that were part of government medical colleges. By 1992 twenty-two such centres were in operation. Most of the 1,300 private hospitals lacked sophisticated medical facilities, although in 1992 approximately 12% possessed state-of-the-art equipment for diagnosis and treatment of all major diseases, including cancer.

The fast pace of development of the private medical sector and the burgeoning middle class in the 1990s have led to the emergence of the new concept in India of establishing hospitals and health care facilities on a for-profit basis.

By the late 1980s, there were approximately 128 medical colleges - roughly three times more than in 1950. These medical colleges in 1987 accepted a combined annual class of 14,166 students. Data for 1987 show that there were 320,000 registered medical practitioners and 219,300 registered nurses. Various studies have shown that in both urban and rural areas people preferred to pay and seek the more sophisticated services provided by private physicians rather than use free treatment at public health centres.

Indigenous or traditional medical practitioners continue to practice throughout the country. The two main forms of traditional medicine practised are the ayurvedic system, which deals with mental and spiritual as well as physical well-being, and the unani (or Galenic) herbal medical practice. A *vaidya* is a practitioner of the ayurvedic tradition, and a *hakim* is a practitioner of the unani or Greek tradition.

These professions are frequently hereditary. A variety of institutions offer training in indigenous medical practice. Only in the late 1970s did official health policy refer to any form of integration between European-trained medical personnel and indigenous medical practitioners. In the early 1990s, there were ninety-eight ayurvedic colleges and seventeen unani colleges operating in both the governmental and non-governmental sectors.

Health Insurance

The majority of the Indian population is unable to access high quality healthcare provided by private players as a result of high costs. Many are now looking towards insurance companies for providing alternative financing options so that they too may seek better quality healthcare. The opportunity remains huge for insurance providers entering into the Indian healthcare market since75% of expenditure on healthcare in India is still being met by 'out-of-pocket' consumers. Even though only 10% of the Indian population today has health insurance coverage, this industry is expected to face tremendous growth over the next few years as a result of several private players that have entered into the market. Health insurance coverage among urban, middle- and upper-class Indians, however, is significantly higher and stands at approximately 50%. The Insurance Regulatory and Development Authority (IRDA) is the governing body responsible for promoting insurance business and introducing insurance regulations in India. The share of public sector companies in health insurance premiums was 76% and that of private sector companies was 24% for the period 2005-06. Health insurance premiums collected over 2005-06 registered a growth of 35% over the previous year. In 2001 the IRDA introduced provisions for Third Party Administrators (TPAs) to support the administration and management of health insurance products offered by insurance companies. TPAs are facilitators in the coordination process between the health insurance provider and the hospital. Currently there are 27 TPAs registered under the IRDA.

Health insurance has a way of increasing accessibility to quality healthcare delivery especially for private healthcare providers for whom high cost remains a barrier. In order to encourage foreign health insurers to enter the Indian market the government has recently proposed to raise the foreign direct investment (FDI) limit in insurance from 26% to 49%. Increasing health insurance penetration and ensuring affordable premium rates are necessary to drive the health insurance market in India.

Medical Tourism

India is becoming a location for medical tourists seeking health care at lower costs than in other countries.

Rate of Growth

India has approximately 600,000 allopathic doctors registered to practice medicine. This number however, is higher than the actual number practicing because it includes doctors who have emigrated to other countries as well as doctors who have died. India licenses 18,000 new doctors a year.

Index

K

L

M

N

O

P

Q

R

S

T

U

V

W

□□□